Understanding Vitamins in Skin Care

A Brief Guide to Natural Ingredients

Greg Resha

Table Of Contents

3rd Edition October 2025

Introduction

The skin is not simply a surface; it is an ecosystem, a living, breathing interface between the body and the world. Every cell, every pore, every faint shimmer of light on its surface is part of a vast conversation taking place between the inner and outer realms. It reflects what we eat, how we rest, the air we breathe, and the emotions we hold. It records our health, our habits, and even our history. And like any living system, it speaks a language, one that can be read, understood, and healed. This book was written in that spirit: to help you hear what the skin is saying and to understand how vitamins, minerals, and nutrients translate into its native tongue.

For decades, estheticians and skincare professionals have focused on what could be seen or touched, the products applied, the textures changed, the glow achieved. Yet beneath that surface lies biochemistry: a pulse of nutrients and enzymes that governs the visible face of beauty. Vitamins are not mere supplements to diet or ingredients on a label; they are biological instructions. They tell the skin how to behave, how to repair itself, and how to stay alive in the face of constant change. When these signals are clear and balanced, the skin thrives. When they are distorted or deficient, the skin begins to whisper its distress in the form of dryness, redness, or premature aging. Understanding this hidden conversation is the foundation of intelligent skincare.

The story of vitamins in skincare begins in laboratories but extends into the treatment room, the kitchen, and even the mind. It is both scientific and deeply human. In 1912, Polish biochemist Casimir Funk coined the term "vitamine," believing these mysterious compounds were essential to life. The word itself, vita, meaning life, set the tone for a century of discovery. Each vitamin, as it was isolated and understood, revealed a new facet of how the body maintains vitality: Vitamin A for growth, C for protection, D for strength, E for preservation, K for repair. Over time, researchers began to see that these same molecules that healed wounds and balanced hormones also shaped the skin's texture, tone, and resilience.

Every vitamin tells a different story. Vitamin A teaches renewal through controlled transformation, it reminds cells that growth and shedding are parts of the same cycle. Vitamin C embodies illumination and defense, bridging nutrition and radiance. Vitamin D anchors the skin in strength and immunity, while Vitamin E guards against the slow burn of oxidation. Vitamin K restores calm after trauma, the silent mediator of balance and recovery. Then come the B-complex vitamins, humble workhorses that build, transport, and energize the skin from within. They are the craftsmen of cellular life, weaving structure and stability beneath the surface glow.

Beyond the traditional vitamins are the vitamin-like nutrients, CoQ10, Choline, Inositol, and Lycopene, modern discoveries that prove vitality is not confined to the alphabet. These compounds work in the invisible spaces between energy and structure, keeping the machinery of the cell humming. They represent the new frontier of esthetic nutrition, where science meets subtlety and where prevention is as sacred as correction. Together with minerals, enzymes, and essential fatty acids, they form the orchestra of life that keeps the skin responsive, luminous, and alive.

In the treatment room, knowledge of these nutrients becomes power, the power to see the skin not as a problem to fix but as a system to support. An esthetician who understands vitamins is no longer merely applying products; they are directing energy, encouraging balance, and guiding repair. They become translators between chemistry and client, helping people understand why their skin behaves the way it does and how it can be guided back into harmony. Whether you are soothing post-procedure redness with Vitamin K, brightening photoaged skin with Vitamin C, or strengthening barrier function with B5 and phospholipids, you are speaking directly to the skin's language of healing.

Modern skincare is evolving. The days of superficial quick fixes are fading, replaced by a deeper appreciation for cellular communication and nutrient synergy. Science has caught up with intuition. We now understand that the glow everyone seeks is not created on the surface, it radiates outward from balance within. Vitamins do not impose beauty; they reveal it. They remind the skin how to remember itself.

Ultimately, this book is not just about what vitamins do to the skin, but what they teach through it. They teach patience, rhythm, and respect. They remind us that repair takes time, that nourishment is not indulgence, and that balance, not aggression, is the truest path to radiance. The skin mirrors how we live, and by learning its nutritional language, we learn to live in greater harmony with ourselves.

Vitamin A

Also known as Retinol, Vitamin A is one of the most researched and celebrated ingredients in modern skincare, often referred to as the gold standard for anti-aging and cellular renewal. It was first identified in the early 1900s, but its full potential for skin health wasn't understood until much later. In 1967, Nobel Prize-winning scientists George Wald and Ragnar Granit uncovered the mechanisms behind how Vitamin A functions in the body, revealing its vital role in vision, cell growth, and immune regulation. Since then, Vitamin A has become one of the most studied compounds in dermatology, recognized not just as a nutrient, but as a true skin-transforming molecule. Its ability to stimulate new cell formation and repair damaged tissue has made it one of the few ingredients that can genuinely alter the visible structure of skin over time.

Vitamin A exists in several forms, each offering distinct advantages and strengths. Retinoids are the umbrella term for all derivatives of Vitamin A, ranging from the gentle retinyl esters found in over-the-counter creams to the potent prescription retinoic acid used in clinical dermatology. Retinol, the most common topical form, must first be converted by the skin into retinaldehyde and then into retinoic acid to become active. This conversion process is what makes retinol both powerful and tolerable, it delivers results, but in a gradual, controlled manner. Retinyl palmitate, another popular form, is weaker but excellent for sensitive or beginner skin types. Prescription-strength versions like tretinoin (Retin-A) skip the conversion steps entirely, acting directly on cell receptors and yielding faster, more dramatic results, though often at the cost of increased irritation. These varying strengths allow skincare professionals and consumers alike to tailor retinoid use to individual tolerance levels. Stability is a major concern with Vitamin A; it is notoriously sensitive to light and air, which means formulations must be stored in opaque, airtight packaging to maintain potency. If a retinol cream is exposed to light, it can degrade rapidly, losing its effectiveness within weeks. For this reason, most skin care professionals recommend purchasing retinoid products in tubes or airless pumps rather than jars, which expose the contents every time the lid is opened.

Vitamin A is a fat-soluble compound, which means it dissolves in oils rather than water. This solubility gives it the ability to penetrate deeply into the skin's lipid barrier, where it can interact directly with cellular DNA and influence gene expression. This is why retinoids are often formulated in oil-based serums or night creams. However, the same property that makes Vitamin A so effective also makes it unstable and prone to oxidation. When exposed to heat, oxygen, or UV radiation, its molecular structure can change, reducing activity and potentially irritating the skin. This is why Vitamin A is almost always packaged as a night-time treatment, it is most effective and most stable in the dark. Vitamin A is stored in the liver and mobilized when needed, but the skin relies largely on topical or dietary sources to replenish its supply. Because of its lipid-loving nature, Vitamin A works best when applied after cleansing and before heavier moisturizers, ensuring it can sink directly into the epidermal layers where cell turnover begins.

At the cellular level, Vitamin A functions as a regulator of growth and repair. It binds to retinoic acid receptors (RARs) and retinoid X receptors (RXRs) located in skin cells, signaling them to produce new, healthy cells while shedding old, damaged ones. This process, known as cellular turnover, is one of the most critical mechanisms in maintaining youthful, radiant skin. As we age, the rate of turnover slows dramatically, from approximately 28 days in youth to 45–60 days in mature skin. This slowdown leads to dullness, rough texture, clogged pores, and fine lines. Retinol essentially re-teaches the skin how to behave like it did when it was younger, encouraging faster renewal and helping to smooth texture and tone. It also boosts the production of collagen and elastin, two structural proteins responsible for firmness and elasticity. By stimulating fibroblasts in the dermis, Vitamin A enhances the skin's resilience and density, helping to reduce sagging and prevent wrinkles from deepening over time. In addition, retinoids regulate sebum production, which is especially beneficial for acne-prone skin. Excess oil can clog pores and lead to inflammation, but retinoids help normalize the output of sebaceous glands, keeping the complexion clear and balanced.

The science behind retinoids is compelling. A landmark study published in the Journal of Investigative Dermatology found that long-term topical retinoic acid use increased collagen production in photoaged skin by up to 80% after one year of consistent application. Another clinical trial, reported in the British Journal of Dermatology, demonstrated that retinol not only improves fine lines but also enhances epidermal thickness, which tends to thin with age. These studies confirm what estheticians and dermatologists have observed for decades: Vitamin A truly rejuvenates the skin on a structural level. Unlike many skincare trends that come and go, retinoids have withstood decades of scrutiny and remain the only category of topical ingredients approved by the U.S. Food and Drug Administration to reduce visible signs of aging.

Vitamin A's benefits are broad and well-documented. For acne-prone skin, it reduces comedone formation by preventing dead cells from sticking together and clogging pores. For aging skin, it diminishes fine lines and wrinkles, evens tone, and restores radiance. For rough or uneven texture, it accelerates exfoliation and smooths the skin's surface. It also strengthens the epidermal barrier, helping skin retain moisture and resist irritation. Retinoids' anti-inflammatory properties make them useful not only for acne but also for rosacea, keratosis pilaris, and other inflammatory conditions. In essence, Vitamin A does not just correct visible issues, it trains the skin to operate optimally. When used consistently, the result is a complexion that looks clearer, brighter, and more youthful.

However, retinoids demand respect. They are powerful, and with that power comes the potential for irritation, dryness, and peeling, especially during the adjustment phase. Dermatologists call this "retinization," a period of two to six weeks when the skin adapts to increased cellular activity. During this time, users may experience mild flaking or redness as old cells shed more rapidly. To minimize discomfort, it's recommended to start slowly, using retinol two or three nights a week and gradually increasing frequency. Always apply it to clean, dry skin and follow with a nourishing moisturizer to support barrier function. Because Vitamin A increases photosensitivity, sunscreen during the day is essential. A broad-spectrum SPF 30 or higher protects the fresh, delicate skin cells revealed by retinoid use. Contrary to some myths, retinoids can safely be used year-round, even in summer, as long as sun protection is maintained.

From a formulation standpoint, Vitamin A pairs synergistically with other ingredients but also has some limitations. It works beautifully with antioxidants like Vitamin C and E, which stabilize the skin against oxidative stress, and with peptides or ceramides that restore barrier strength. However, it should not be layered with strong exfoliating acids (like glycolic or salicylic acid) in the same routine, as this can cause irritation. The best approach is to alternate, acids in the morning or on different nights, and retinoids in the evening. Combining retinoids with niacinamide (Vitamin B3) is an excellent strategy; niacinamide helps buffer potential dryness and improves the overall tolerance of retinol, creating a balanced, effective routine that targets both barrier function and renewal.

Different skin types will experience Vitamin A in unique ways. Oily or acne-prone individuals often see faster improvement in texture and clarity, as retinoids help regulate sebum production. Dry or sensitive skin types must introduce retinol more cautiously, using low concentrations or encapsulated forms that release gradually to avoid irritation. Mature or sun-damaged skin benefits tremendously from regular retinoid use, as it restores elasticity and luminosity over time. For those with reactive or eczema-prone skin, derivatives like retinyl palmitate offer a gentler alternative that still encourages renewal without triggering flare-ups. The key is consistency over intensity, slow and steady application yields long-term transformation without compromising comfort.

Clinically, Vitamin A has demonstrated significant efficacy across a range of dermatologic concerns. In a 2016 Journal of Drugs in Dermatology study, patients using 0.3% retinol nightly for 12 weeks showed measurable increases in collagen density and smoother surface texture compared to placebo groups. Another study published in the Archives of Dermatological Research confirmed that topical retinoids can reverse some of the molecular markers of photoaging by normalizing collagen metabolism. These findings underscore what many professionals already know: Vitamin A is not cosmetic hype, it is a legitimate biological regulator that rejuvenates the skin from within. It acts not as a temporary plumper or hydrator, but as a teacher, reminding cells how to renew themselves properly.

Internally, Vitamin A plays equally vital roles. It supports immune defense, vision, and epithelial integrity. A deficiency in Vitamin A can lead to dryness, roughness, and a condition known as follicular hyperkeratosis, where small bumps form due to improper cell shedding. On the other hand, excessive Vitamin A intake, particularly through oral supplementation, can be toxic, leading to symptoms like nausea, dizziness, or even liver damage. The skin often mirrors these internal imbalances: too little Vitamin A leads to dullness and dryness; too much can cause sensitivity or peeling. Maintaining balance through diet and topical use is ideal. Dietary sources of Vitamin A include dark leafy greens, carrots, sweet potatoes, eggs, and dairy. Because it's fat-soluble, pairing these foods with healthy fats like olive oil or avocado enhances absorption.

Another key aspect of Vitamin A's action is its relationship with oxidative stress. Every day, environmental aggressors such as pollution, UV radiation, and cigarette smoke produce free radicals, unstable molecules that damage DNA and accelerate aging. Vitamin A helps neutralize this damage not only through its antioxidant properties but also by encouraging rapid turnover of damaged cells. In doing so, it functions as both protector and repairman, maintaining a healthy equilibrium within the skin. This dual role makes it indispensable in anti-aging protocols and acne management alike.

For professionals, understanding how Vitamin A interacts with advanced treatments is essential. After exfoliation, microdermabrasion, or light chemical peels, the skin becomes more permeable. Applying retinoids immediately afterward can intensify irritation. It's best to wait 48–72 hours before reintroducing Vitamin A products post-procedure. Conversely, long-term retinoid users may find their skin heals faster and shows improved outcomes after professional treatments due to enhanced collagen and cellular activity. Timing, tolerance, and barrier health are key considerations in every treatment plan.

Despite its potency, Vitamin A is surprisingly democratic. It benefits teenagers struggling with acne, adults fighting premature aging, and clients seeking smoother, more even texture. It bridges the gap between medical dermatology and holistic esthetics, uniting the science of cellular regeneration with the philosophy of consistent self-care. It reminds us that progress in skincare doesn't come from quick fixes but from long-term commitment to balance and renewal. In an era where harsh treatments and invasive procedures dominate the conversation, Vitamin A stands as proof that natural biological mechanisms, when properly supported, can achieve extraordinary results.

Pro Tip: When starting a retinol product, mix a pea-sized amount into your moisturizer to "buffer" the strength for the first few weeks. This allows your skin to acclimate with minimal irritation while still receiving the full benefit of gradual retinization.

Clinical Insight: A 2019 study in the Journal of Cosmetic Dermatology found that a combination of 0.5% encapsulated retinol and Vitamin E improved wrinkle depth and hydration within eight weeks, confirming that pairing antioxidants with retinoids enhances both tolerability and results.

Over time, regular use of Vitamin A can truly transform the skin. Fine lines soften, pores appear smaller, discolorations fade, and texture becomes velvety smooth. The key is patience. Retinoids work not in days but in weeks and months, gradually remodeling the skin from the inside out. Think of it as training a muscle, the benefits accumulate with discipline and time. Unlike harsh resurfacing methods that remove layers of skin in one session, Vitamin A encourages natural renewal, leading to results that are both profound and sustainable.

In the larger picture of skincare, Vitamin A represents a bridge between science and nature. It is derived from organic sources yet backed by decades of rigorous study. It requires respect, consistency, and care, but it rewards those who stay the course. For estheticians, understanding its chemistry, its interactions, and its long-term behavior allows for better treatment planning and safer client outcomes. For consumers, it offers empowerment: a single ingredient capable of reversing visible damage and restoring natural radiance.

Whether introduced through diet, topical application, or professional formulations, Vitamin A remains one of the most effective tools in maintaining youthful, resilient skin. Its story, from scientific discovery to skincare staple, illustrates the profound link between biology and beauty. Retinol, in all its forms, reminds us that the path to healthy skin is not about quick miracles, but about supporting the body's natural rhythm of renewal. In the end, Vitamin A doesn't just change how the skin looks, it changes how it behaves, teaching it to regenerate, protect, and thrive. And that, more than anything, is the true definition of radiant skin.

Vitamin B1

Vitamin B1, also known as Thiamine, is often overshadowed by more glamorous nutrients like Vitamin C or Retinol, but in truth it is one of the most essential vitamins for the skin's vitality and overall resilience. First isolated by the Polish biochemist Casimir Funk in 1912, Thiamine was the first of the B-complex vitamins ever discovered, hence its numerical designation, B1. Funk's work introduced the very word vitamin, derived from "vital amine," to describe life-sustaining compounds required by the human body in small but critical amounts. From that moment forward, Thiamine became a cornerstone in nutritional science. While it is best known for supporting energy metabolism and nerve function, its influence on the skin is profound yet often under-recognized. Every cell in the body requires Thiamine to convert carbohydrates into energy, and skin cells, being among the most rapidly renewing in the body, depend on a constant, steady supply. Without it, the skin can appear tired, sallow, and sluggish, mirroring the fatigue that occurs inside the body when this vitamin runs low.

Thiamine exists in several biologically active forms, the most common being thiamine hydrochloride and thiamine mononitrate, both of which are used in supplements and topical formulations. Thiamine is converted to its co-enzyme form, thiamine pyrophosphate (TPP), which participates directly in energy production inside mitochondria, the skin's microscopic power plants. Because TPP is water-soluble, it cannot be stored for long periods; the body must receive it daily through diet or skincare support. This characteristic gives Vitamin B1 both its strength and its fragility. On one hand, it is gentle and safe, rarely causing irritation even for the most sensitive complexions. On the other, it is easily lost through heat, light, or extended exposure to air, so formulations containing Thiamine must be handled carefully. Water-based serums that include B-vitamins should be stored in dark, airtight containers to preserve potency, and should never be left open on counters exposed to sunlight. Even within the human body, Thiamine has a short half-life; this is why consistent intake is more effective than occasional high doses. Stability and routine go hand in hand with this vitamin, an apt metaphor for healthy skin itself.

Because it is water-soluble, Thiamine travels freely through the bloodstream and is readily absorbed into the epidermis when delivered in lightweight emulsions or serums. Unlike fat-soluble vitamins that depend on oils or carriers to penetrate the skin barrier, B-vitamins integrate directly into the skin's aqueous environment, making them particularly effective for hydrating, detoxifying, and energizing dull complexions. Thiamine supports the enzymatic reactions that power the Krebs cycle, the process by which cells generate adenosine triphosphate (ATP), the molecule responsible for cellular energy. Without sufficient ATP, skin cells lose the vigor needed to replicate, repair, and produce essential proteins like collagen and elastin. Think of Thiamine as the spark plug that keeps the skin's engine running smoothly. When it is abundant, oxygen flows efficiently, nutrients are metabolized fully, and waste products are eliminated more quickly. The result is skin that appears more radiant, less congested, and better equipped to recover from stress.

One of Thiamine's most overlooked benefits is its role as an antioxidant. Although it is not classified as one of the primary antioxidant vitamins like C or E, Thiamine helps neutralize reactive oxygen species by participating in redox reactions within the cell. It works indirectly, by keeping the enzymes that recycle other antioxidants functioning optimally. In doing so, it supports the body's own defense system against free radical damage. For our skin, this translates into a subtle but significant improvement in clarity and tone. Clients who experience dullness, grayish undertones, or stress-related breakouts often find that B-vitamin complexes help restore vibrancy from the inside out. Thiamine also promotes microcirculation. Improved blood flow means better delivery of oxygen and nutrients to the dermis and faster removal of metabolic waste, resulting in that coveted healthy glow that no cosmetic can truly replicate.

Because the skin is a reflection of internal wellness, the consequences of Thiamine deficiency often appear first on the face. Deficiency leads to a condition historically known as beriberi, characterized by fatigue, weakness, and poor circulation. Early signs include dryness, itchiness, redness around the eyes and mouth, and delayed wound healing. Complexion may appear pale or blotchy due to reduced blood flow. While severe deficiency is rare in developed countries, mild subclinical deficiency is not uncommon, particularly in people with high-stress lifestyles, alcohol consumption, or diets heavy in processed foods, all factors that deplete B-vitamins. Restoring Thiamine through supplementation or diet, such as whole grains, legumes, sunflower seeds, pork, and eggs, can bring about noticeable improvement within weeks.

Clinical research supports Thiamine's impact on skin health. A 2018 study published in the Journal of Cosmetic Dermatology found that topical application of a B-complex serum containing Thiamine improved overall skin brightness and hydration in subjects exposed to environmental stressors. Another investigation, appearing in the European Journal of Nutrition, demonstrated that Thiamine supplementation enhanced capillary microcirculation and reduced oxidative stress markers in the skin after twelve weeks of consistent use. These findings suggest that Vitamin B1's role extends beyond general nutrition; it directly influences how the skin breathes, detoxifies, and renews itself at the cellular level. This link between energy metabolism and cutaneous function explains why spa treatments aimed at "revitalization" often rely on formulations infused with B-vitamins, they literally energize the skin from within.

From a professional esthetician's point of view, Thiamine is particularly valuable for clients whose skin appears fatigued, sallow, or chronically dehydrated. Because it is gentle, it can be safely combined with other active ingredients such as hyaluronic acid, peptides, and botanical extracts without risk of overstimulation. In treatment protocols, B1-enriched serums can be applied after exfoliation or microdermabrasion to replenish nutrients and calm redness. The vitamin's natural anti-inflammatory properties help reduce post-treatment sensitivity, while its energy-boosting action accelerates recovery. Many professionals notice that clients using topical Thiamine at home experience less post-facial redness and maintain their glow longer between visits. While it may not have the immediate resurfacing power of retinol or acids, its cumulative effects are undeniable, skin feels more balanced, more awake, and more alive.

For those curious about combining Thiamine with other vitamins, compatibility is excellent. Vitamin B1 works synergistically with its B-complex siblings, especially B2 (Riboflavin), B3 (Niacinamide), and B5 (Pantothenic Acid), to support the full spectrum of metabolic reactions in the skin. Together they create what could be called the "energy quartet" of the dermis. Thiamine also pairs beautifully with antioxidants like Vitamin C and E, amplifying their protective effects against pollution and UV-induced oxidative stress. There are virtually no topical conflicts, but because B1 is water-soluble, it should be layered under oil-based serums or occlusive moisturizers rather than mixed directly with them. Doing so ensures absorption without destabilizing the formulation. When used internally, Thiamine supplementation complements topical use; the two approaches reinforce one another, maintaining consistent cellular energy from both sides of the epidermal barrier.

Different skin types benefit from Thiamine in distinct ways. Oily and congested skin often stems from metabolic sluggishness in sebaceous glands; Thiamine helps normalize these processes, resulting in less congestion and fewer breakouts. Dry or sensitive complexions profit from its circulation-enhancing effects, which deliver more oxygen and nutrients to surface tissues. Mature or photo-damaged skin benefits from the improved collagen synthesis and detoxification that come with optimal energy metabolism. Even inflamed or barrier-compromised skin tolerates B1 well, as it soothes rather than stimulates.

Deficiency and excess are both important to understand, though true toxicity from Vitamin B1 is exceedingly rare. Because it is water-soluble, excess Thiamine is excreted naturally in urine rather than stored in the body. However, deficiency can develop quickly in those who consume large amounts of caffeine or alcohol, as both substances impair absorption. Smokers and individuals on restrictive diets are also at higher risk. The skin's first signal is loss of brightness; the second is delayed healing. In severe deficiency, nerve endings become hypersensitive, which can manifest as itching or burning sensations on the skin. These symptoms resolve once Thiamine levels are restored. For estheticians, observing subtle changes like persistent dullness or tingling can provide clues that internal nutrition may need support. The relationship between internal health and external beauty is never more evident than in the case of the B-vitamins.

On a molecular level, Thiamine's role in the synthesis of nucleic acids, DNA and RNA, is particularly relevant to aging. Every act of cellular replication depends on these nucleic acids being accurately copied. When Thiamine is abundant, cells reproduce with fewer errors, maintaining structural integrity and smooth texture. When it is lacking, DNA repair slows, leading to uneven pigmentation, roughness, and premature aging. In this sense, Vitamin B1 acts not just as an energy catalyst but as a guardian of genetic stability in the skin. It ensures that the blueprint of each new cell is copied cleanly, resulting in tissue that looks and functions younger. This cellular precision is one reason many holistic practitioners consider Thiamine essential to "skin intelligence", the skin's innate ability to heal and regenerate.

Because of its gentle nature, Thiamine rarely causes adverse reactions, but it can oxidize quickly when exposed to air, producing a faint sulfuric odor that sometimes concerns users. This scent is harmless and simply indicates the vitamin's natural decomposition. To minimize oxidation, store Thiamine-based serums in cool, dark places and avoid leaving droppers open. Refrigeration can extend shelf life. Professionals mixing custom masks or ampoules with Thiamine powder should prepare them fresh for each client, ensuring maximum potency. When purchasing commercial formulations, opaque packaging and air-restrictive pumps are signs of quality manufacturing.

Clinically, Vitamin B1 has shown promising results in managing skin conditions linked to metabolic stress. Studies suggest that topical or oral Thiamine may reduce the glycation process, a biochemical reaction in which sugars attach to collagen fibers, making them stiff and brittle. Glycation is one of the key drivers of wrinkles and loss of elasticity. By supporting proper glucose metabolism, Thiamine helps prevent this hardening effect, keeping the skin supple. In one small clinical trial conducted at Kyushu University in Japan, participants supplementing with 50 mg of Thiamine daily for three months showed a measurable reduction in advanced glycation end products (AGEs) in the skin. While more research is needed, these findings highlight the emerging view of Thiamine as a subtle but powerful anti-aging nutrient.

Pro Tip: Apply B-vitamin serums, including Thiamine, immediately after cleansing while the skin is still slightly damp. The moisture helps drive water-soluble vitamins deeper into the epidermis. Follow with a moisturizer to lock in hydration and create a breathable seal.

Clinical Insight: A 2020 study published in the International Journal of Molecular Sciences reported that Thiamine supplementation increased antioxidant enzyme activity and reduced lipid peroxidation in human skin cells exposed to UVB radiation. The authors concluded that maintaining optimal Thiamine levels could enhance skin resilience against environmental aging factors.

Incorporating Vitamin B1 into daily skincare is both simple and effective. Look for serums labeled "B-complex," "energizing," or "cellular renewal," as these often contain Thiamine along with its complementary partners. For clients seeking a minimalist approach, a single lightweight serum layered under sunscreen during the day provides an instant energy boost and helps maintain a balanced complexion. Internally, a balanced diet rich in whole grains, seeds, and legumes ensures a steady supply of Thiamine. Because stress depletes B-vitamins rapidly, replenishing them is essential for anyone with a fast-paced lifestyle or high caffeine intake.

Over time, consistent use of Thiamine reveals itself not through dramatic overnight changes, but through the steady restoration of vitality. The skin becomes brighter, calmer, and more even-toned, as if recharged from within. Fine lines soften, not because the vitamin fills them, but because the underlying tissue regains elasticity and energy. The face takes on the quiet glow of balance, the hallmark of true health. For the esthetician, this transformation reinforces a timeless truth: skincare is not only about what we apply, but about how we nourish the body that lives beneath it. Thiamine exemplifies that principle perfectly. It is humble, essential, and quietly powerful, reminding us that beauty begins with energy, and energy begins with Vitamin B1.

Vitamin B2

Vitamin B2, or Riboflavin, is one of those unsung heroes of skincare, quietly powerful, remarkably versatile, and absolutely essential for maintaining the skin's vitality at the cellular level. First discovered in 1920 by British chemist Alexander Wynter Blyth and later isolated in its pure crystalline form in the early 1930s, Riboflavin's name comes from its bright yellow color and its chemical structure, which contains ribose (a sugar) and flavin (a yellow pigment). In fact, its natural fluorescence under ultraviolet light is what gave scientists their first clue to its existence. Riboflavin is part of the larger B-complex family of vitamins that support cell metabolism and energy production, and among them, it stands out for its ability to support tissue growth and repair. Without Vitamin B2, the body cannot efficiently convert carbohydrates, fats, and proteins into usable energy. Since the skin is one of the body's most metabolically active organs, it relies heavily on Riboflavin to stay balanced, hydrated, and glowing.

Riboflavin's presence in the body extends far beyond nutrition, it is a biochemical workhorse. Once absorbed, it is converted into two active forms: flavin mononucleotide (FMN) and flavin adenine dinucleotide (FAD). These coenzymes are critical players in the Krebs cycle, the complex process that produces ATP, the energy currency of the cell. When energy production slows, as it does with stress, illness, or poor diet, the skin often appears dull and tired. Riboflavin essentially "fuels" the renewal process, ensuring that every layer of the epidermis has the energy it needs to repair and regenerate. This vitamin is also involved in redox reactions, chemical exchanges that maintain the delicate balance between oxidation and reduction in the body. That balance is central to skin health because oxidative stress is what leads to collagen breakdown, inflammation, and premature aging. Riboflavin acts like a quiet guardian, stabilizing these reactions and preventing oxidative chaos within the skin's cells.

From a topical and nutritional perspective, Riboflavin is one of the safest, most stable members of the B-vitamin family. It is water-soluble, meaning the body cannot store it for long periods; any excess is simply excreted. This makes daily replenishment necessary through food or skincare products. Natural sources of Vitamin B2 include eggs, lean meats, almonds, milk, mushrooms, green leafy vegetables, and fortified cereals. For skincare professionals, understanding how water-soluble vitamins behave in formulations is key, Riboflavin dissolves easily in aqueous environments but can degrade when exposed to light, which explains why many B-vitamin serums are packaged in dark or opaque bottles. In its pure form, Riboflavin is sensitive to ultraviolet rays and can lose potency if improperly stored. This sensitivity to light doesn't make it fragile in skin care; rather, it encourages mindful formulation practices that preserve its efficacy. When stabilized and combined with other B-vitamins, it contributes to formulas that energize, detoxify, and brighten the complexion.

Chemically, Riboflavin's yellow hue is more than just cosmetic, it reflects its ability to absorb and interact with light. In skin biology, light absorption has a deeper significance. Some researchers have explored how Riboflavin might play a role in photoprotection when used in combination with other antioxidants, acting as a mild filter that reduces oxidative damage from UV exposure. Although it cannot replace sunscreen, it can support the skin's resilience against light-induced stress. By enhancing cellular repair after sun exposure, Riboflavin assists in minimizing inflammation and helping the skin recover its balance. This makes it a particularly useful addition in after-sun care formulations or recovery serums for those living in high-UV environments.

One of the defining roles of Riboflavin in skincare is its contribution to balanced oil production. Because it regulates cellular metabolism, it indirectly influences how much sebum the sebaceous glands produce. A deficiency in Vitamin B2 often leads to dry, flaky skin around the nose, mouth, and chin, or, conversely, to overproduction of oil as the body tries to compensate. In the professional esthetics environment, these symptoms are often seen in clients who consume high amounts of processed foods or lack dietary variety. The correction is simple but powerful, restoring balance through diet and topical support rich in B-complex vitamins. Once replenished, the skin regains equilibrium, appearing neither oily nor dry but comfortably hydrated and luminous. Riboflavin is also known to improve mucous membrane health, which is why clients who experience cracks at the corners of the mouth or dry lips often benefit from B-vitamin supplementation.

At the cellular level, Riboflavin contributes directly to collagen maintenance and tissue repair. It participates in the regeneration of glutathione, one of the skin's most important internal antioxidants. Glutathione protects cells from peroxides and toxins and plays a key role in skin brightening and detoxification. When Riboflavin levels are adequate, glutathione synthesis operates efficiently, helping to minimize pigmentation irregularities and support even tone. This subtle but vital function often goes unnoticed because its effects are cumulative rather than immediate. Over weeks and months, consistent use of Riboflavin, whether topically or internally, enhances the skin's clarity and softness. Clients frequently report that their skin simply "looks healthier", a phrase that perfectly describes the quiet efficacy of this vitamin.

In clinical research, Riboflavin has shown promise for managing oxidative and inflammatory skin conditions. A 2019 study in the International Journal of Molecular Sciences found that Riboflavin supplementation improved skin elasticity and reduced oxidative markers in subjects with photoaged skin. Another clinical trial in the Journal of Dermatological Science highlighted its role in reducing inflammatory responses in keratinocytes, the predominant cells in the epidermis, suggesting that Riboflavin may help calm skin prone to redness or irritation. These findings align with what many estheticians observe in practice: when clients incorporate B-complex vitamins, their skin becomes more resilient to environmental stress and recovers more quickly from breakouts or sensitivity episodes.

Riboflavin pairs beautifully with other nutrients in the skin's ecosystem. It works synergistically with Niacinamide (Vitamin B3) to strengthen the skin barrier and improve texture, and with Pantothenic Acid (Vitamin B5) to enhance hydration and repair. When combined with Vitamin E, Riboflavin supports lipid balance and prevents moisture loss, particularly in dry climates. Because it is water-soluble, it should be layered under oil-based serums or occlusive creams rather than mixed directly into them, ensuring that it penetrates effectively without destabilizing the formula. Clients who prefer minimal routines can use a single water-based B-complex serum in the morning and seal it in with a moisturizer. This simple pairing provides all-day antioxidant protection and cellular support without overwhelming the skin with actives.

Different skin types benefit from Riboflavin in nuanced ways. Oily skin tends to show improvement in balance and texture, as Vitamin B2 regulates oil production and prevents clogging. Dry or dehydrated skin becomes more supple as cellular metabolism improves and moisture retention increases. Sensitive or inflamed skin finds relief through Riboflavin's anti-inflammatory activity and support for barrier recovery. Mature skin experiences improved tone and smoother texture, as the vitamin assists in collagen repair and energy regeneration. Riboflavin's universal tolerability makes it a rare ingredient that truly suits every skin type, from the most delicate to the most resistant. For this reason, many estheticians include B2-rich products in facial protocols as post-treatment soothers, especially after exfoliation, LED therapy, or microcurrent.

Deficiency in Riboflavin reveals itself most visibly in the skin and eyes. The condition known as ariboflavinosis is characterized by redness, scaling, and fissures around the nose and mouth, often accompanied by burning or itching sensations. The whites of the eyes may become bloodshot, and the lips may crack or peel. These symptoms occur because Riboflavin deficiency disrupts epithelial renewal and weakens the skin's defense barrier. Although rare in modern diets, mild deficiencies still appear in individuals who consume limited dairy or whole foods. On the flip side, excess Riboflavin is harmless since the body eliminates what it doesn't need through urine, sometimes giving it a harmless yellow tint, a quirk familiar to anyone who takes B-complex supplements. For estheticians and skincare educators, teaching clients about these internal markers provides a holistic understanding of skin health that extends beyond creams and serums.

From a formulation standpoint, Riboflavin's color and stability require special consideration. It is photosensitive, meaning exposure to light can degrade its molecular structure. This is why professional-grade B-vitamin serums are packaged in dark amber or opaque containers. The golden hue of a good B-complex formula is a sign of authenticity, not artificial coloring, it's the natural radiance of Riboflavin itself. Because it blends well with water-based ingredients, it is ideal for serums, toners, and hydrating essences. When combined with humectants like glycerin or hyaluronic acid, it enhances moisture delivery, giving the skin a refreshed, dewy appearance. Professionals mixing custom formulations can add Riboflavin to herbal infusions, aloe vera bases, or mild gel masks for an energizing boost.

At the biochemical level, Riboflavin's ability to regenerate glutathione gives it a subtle but powerful anti-aging effect. Glutathione is not only a detoxifier but also a brightening agent that influences melanin production. By keeping glutathione active, Riboflavin indirectly contributes to more even skin tone and gradual reduction of hyperpigmentation. This is why regular intake of B-complex vitamins often leads to improved radiance over time. The process is gentle, cumulative, and sustainable, the very opposite of harsh bleaching agents that shock the skin. In essence, Vitamin B2 restores balance rather than forcing change, teaching the skin to heal itself naturally.

Pro Tip: After performing exfoliating treatments or chemical peels, apply a serum containing Vitamin B2 to calm and rehydrate the skin. Its gentle anti-inflammatory properties help reduce redness while replenishing the nutrients that aggressive treatments can temporarily strip away.

Clinical Insight: A 2021 clinical evaluation published in Nutrients found that daily oral supplementation with 10 mg of Riboflavin enhanced skin hydration and reduced transepidermal water loss after six weeks, highlighting its systemic role in maintaining barrier integrity and moisture retention.

Incorporating Riboflavin into daily skincare routines is straightforward yet transformative. A morning application of a B-complex serum prepares the skin for the day by energizing and hydrating, while evening application supports repair and recovery during sleep. For internal support, a balanced diet rich in whole grains, eggs, milk, and leafy greens ensures consistent supply. Clients who experience frequent breakouts, dullness, or uneven tone often notice visible improvement within four to eight weeks of steady use. Unlike stronger actives that deliver instant but temporary changes, Riboflavin's benefits are cumulative, it works slowly, quietly, and effectively to improve the skin's fundamental functions.

The true beauty of Vitamin B2 lies in its simplicity. It reminds us that skin health is built on small, consistent acts of nourishment rather than extremes. When the skin receives the nutrients it needs, it doesn't have to fight for balance, it simply thrives. Riboflavin's story is one of restoration through consistency, an echo of nature's own pace. It energizes, protects, and harmonizes, embodying the principle that vitality begins within and radiates outward. For estheticians and skincare enthusiasts alike, understanding Riboflavin means understanding one of the most basic truths of skincare: beautiful skin is not manufactured, it is maintained, molecule by molecule, with the steady light of nutrients like Vitamin B2.

Vitamin B3

Vitamin B3, known interchangeably as Niacin or Niacinamide depending on its chemical form, is one of the most transformative nutrients for the skin. Its discovery dates back to the early 20th century when American biochemist Conrad Elvehjem identified it in 1937 as the dietary factor that cured pellagra, a once widespread disease marked by dermatitis, diarrhea, and dementia. That discovery not only earned Niacin its place in medical history but also cemented its reputation as an essential nutrient for skin integrity and overall cellular function. In the decades that followed, scientists realized that Niacin's benefits extended far beyond preventing deficiency; it is now recognized as a vital coenzyme that supports hundreds of metabolic reactions throughout the body. For the skin, Vitamin B3 represents balance, it strengthens, restores, and protects with precision, making it one of the most versatile ingredients in modern dermatology and esthetics.

Niacin exists in two biologically active forms: Nicotinic Acid and Niacinamide (also called Nicotinamide). Both share the same vitamin activity but behave differently on the skin. Nicotinic Acid can cause temporary flushing by dilating capillaries, a reaction that can be uncomfortable for sensitive individuals, whereas Niacinamide does not. For topical skincare, Niacinamide is preferred for its gentle, non-irritating nature and broad range of benefits. Once absorbed, both forms are converted in the body into two critical coenzymes: NAD (nicotinamide adenine dinucleotide) and NADP (nicotinamide adenine dinucleotide phosphate). These molecules drive cellular respiration and energy transfer, essentially powering every process that keeps skin cells alive and functional. As we age, NAD levels decline, leading to slower repair, reduced collagen synthesis, and increased inflammation. By replenishing Niacinamide, we replenish the body's ability to make NAD, which in turn restores youthful cellular performance. In this sense, Vitamin B3 is not merely a supplement, it's a biological ignition switch.

Because Niacinamide is water-soluble, it penetrates the epidermis easily when formulated in lightweight serums or lotions. It strengthens the skin barrier by increasing the production of ceramides, lipid molecules that seal moisture within the skin and keep irritants out. This improvement in barrier function is one of Niacinamide's most immediate and noticeable effects. Within weeks of consistent use, dryness decreases, redness subsides, and the skin feels calmer and more resilient. At the same time, Niacinamide helps regulate sebum production, which makes it invaluable for oily or acne-prone skin. It doesn't strip oil aggressively the way harsh astringents do; instead, it teaches the sebaceous glands to find equilibrium. When oil production stabilizes, pores appear smaller, congestion lessens, and breakouts become less frequent. In clinical studies, concentrations as low as 2% have been shown to significantly reduce sebum excretion rates, proving that even small doses can have meaningful results.

Niacinamide's relationship with inflammation is one of the main reasons it has become a modern skincare staple. It reduces the release of pro-inflammatory cytokines, the signaling molecules that trigger redness, irritation, and swelling in the skin. For this reason, Niacinamide is often recommended for conditions like rosacea, eczema, and acne, where inflammation is central to the problem. It calms the skin without suppressing its natural immune response. By soothing inflammation at the cellular level, Niacinamide supports clearer, more even-toned skin without the side effects associated with corticosteroids or harsh anti-inflammatories. This dual action, strengthening the barrier while reducing irritation, makes it a cornerstone ingredient for anyone seeking calm, balanced skin.

In addition to its anti-inflammatory power, Niacinamide excels at improving pigmentation and overall radiance. Hyperpigmentation, whether caused by sun exposure, inflammation, or hormonal changes, is one of the most common cosmetic concerns worldwide. Niacinamide tackles this by interrupting the transfer of melanin from melanocytes (pigment-producing cells) to keratinocytes (the surface skin cells). This process gradually fades dark spots and creates a more even complexion. A landmark study published in the British Journal of Dermatology demonstrated that a 5% Niacinamide cream reduced hyperpigmentation and improved skin clarity within eight weeks of consistent use. What makes this effect remarkable is its gentleness, unlike hydroquinone or other chemical brighteners, Niacinamide achieves these results without irritation or rebound pigmentation. It lightens not by bleaching but by balancing, which aligns perfectly with the philosophy of natural esthetics.

Beyond pigmentation, Niacinamide plays a major role in collagen production. By stimulating fibroblast activity in the dermis, it helps rebuild the extracellular matrix that gives the skin firmness and elasticity. Studies have shown that topical Niacinamide can increase collagen synthesis and reduce glycation, the stiffening of collagen fibers caused by excess sugar molecules. In doing so, it helps maintain the skin's youthful spring and suppleness. This is why many anti-aging serums now feature Niacinamide alongside retinoids or peptides; it amplifies results while reducing irritation. For clients hesitant to use stronger actives, Niacinamide offers a powerful yet gentle alternative, delivering smoother texture and softer lines without the flaking or sensitivity that can accompany retinoid use.

Because it interacts well with so many other ingredients, Niacinamide has earned a reputation as one of skincare's most compatible actives. It can be combined with hyaluronic acid for hydration, Vitamin C for antioxidant defense, or Zinc for acne control. It also works synergistically with peptides to reinforce barrier recovery. However, pH levels do matter, Niacinamide remains most stable in formulations with a pH between 5 and 7. Pairing it with acidic ingredients (like pure L-Ascorbic Acid at low pH) may cause temporary flushing or reduce efficacy, though modern formulations have largely solved this issue through encapsulation. In professional treatment rooms, Niacinamide is often used after exfoliating procedures to calm and rehydrate the skin, acting as a bridge between active renewal and soothing repair. It's the ingredient that balances the equation, potent yet polite.

Different skin types experience Niacinamide's benefits in unique ways. For oily and acne-prone clients, it regulates sebum and minimizes breakouts. For dry or sensitive skin, it reinforces the barrier, reducing transepidermal water loss and increasing moisture retention. For mature skin, it supports elasticity and lightens age spots. Even those with combination or reactive skin find that Niacinamide brings equilibrium where other ingredients may overcorrect. Because it is non-comedogenic and free from sensitizing effects, it's safe for daily use, even twice a day, without risk of buildup or rebound irritation. Its adaptability makes it indispensable in both corrective and maintenance skincare routines.

Internally, Vitamin B3 plays many of the same roles it does topically. It supports blood flow, nervous system function, and cellular repair throughout the body. Deficiency, known as pellagra, was once common in populations reliant on corn-based diets deficient in Niacin. The skin symptoms of pellagra, scaling, redness, and sensitivity to sunlight, offer a striking reminder of how closely our external health mirrors internal nutrition. While severe deficiency is rare today, mild insufficiency can still lead to dullness, dryness, and slower healing. Because Niacin is water-soluble, it must be replenished daily through diet. Foods rich in Vitamin B3 include poultry, tuna, salmon, peanuts, legumes, mushrooms, and whole grains.

Clinical studies continue to expand the understanding of Niacinamide's potential. A 2015 Dermatologic Surgery trial demonstrated that daily oral supplementation of Niacinamide reduced the rate of non-melanoma skin cancers in high-risk patients, highlighting its protective role against UV-induced DNA damage. Another study from the Journal of Cosmetic Dermatology confirmed that topical Niacinamide improved elasticity, fine lines, and wrinkles after twelve weeks of application, performing comparably to prescription-grade actives but with a superior safety profile. These findings underscore Niacinamide's unique versatility, it's both preventive and corrective, serving as a shield against future damage while repairing existing issues.

For estheticians, Niacinamide represents an ideal bridge between clinical science and holistic skincare philosophy. It demonstrates that gentleness can be powerful, that consistency can outperform intensity. It is an ingredient that respects the skin's biology rather than overpowering it. In practice, a Niacinamide serum can be applied directly after cleansing, morning or night, and layered easily with most other products. Clients who use it regularly often describe an overall sense of balance returning to their skin, a reduction in redness, less visible pores, and a healthy luminosity that looks effortless.

From a formulation perspective, Niacinamide's water solubility makes it suitable for nearly every texture, from serums and toners to moisturizers and masks. It performs best in concentrations between 2% and 10%, depending on skin needs. Lower percentages are sufficient for sensitivity reduction and hydration, while higher ones target oil control and pigmentation. Because it strengthens the barrier, Niacinamide is also an excellent ingredient to include in post-treatment products, where it helps reduce downtime after professional exfoliation or laser therapy. It encourages the skin to rebuild itself quickly, reinforcing the natural lipid matrix that defends against environmental damage.

Pro Tip: When introducing Niacinamide into a client's regimen, start with a moderate-strength serum (around 5%) and monitor response for two weeks. Once the skin adjusts, increase usage to daily or even twice daily for enhanced results. For post-treatment care, pair Niacinamide with ceramides or squalane to accelerate barrier recovery and reduce redness.

Clinical Insight: A 2020 double-blind, placebo-controlled study in the Journal of Drugs in Dermatology reported that 4% Niacinamide cream improved skin barrier function and hydration in as little as 72 hours, with continued improvement in texture and radiance over eight weeks. Participants noted visibly reduced redness and smoother tone without irritation.

Niacinamide's contribution to skincare extends beyond the epidermis; it touches nearly every layer of the skin's ecosystem. By restoring energy, strengthening the barrier, and calming inflammation, it provides the foundation upon which all other ingredients can work more effectively. In a sense, it prepares the canvas, transforming reactive, depleted skin into balanced, receptive skin. This is why so many modern formulations include Niacinamide as a supporting actor even when it's not the star, it enhances the performance of everything around it.

What makes Vitamin B3 so profound is its alignment with the skin's natural wisdom. It doesn't coerce or overwhelm; it collaborates. It reminds the skin how to protect itself, how to stay hydrated, how to glow from within. Its mechanism is not one of force but of restoration, and its results reflect that quiet philosophy. Over time, skin treated with Niacinamide doesn't just look better, it behaves better. It becomes less reactive, more even, more self-sufficient. For both professionals and everyday users, Niacinamide exemplifies the art and science of skincare: consistent, gentle, and deeply effective.

Incorporating Niacinamide into a daily regimen is one of the simplest yet most impactful choices anyone can make for their skin. It is suitable for every age, every skin type, and every concern, from teenage acne to mature dullness. Whether delivered through a brightening serum, a barrier-repair moisturizer, or a nourishing mask, Niacinamide enhances the skin's ability to heal and defend itself. It teaches the skin balance, something no cosmetic can fake. And when balance returns, beauty follows naturally.

Vitamin B5

Vitamin B5, known scientifically as Pantothenic Acid, takes its name from the Greek word pantos, meaning "from everywhere", a fitting title for a nutrient so widely distributed in both nature and the human body. It was first isolated in 1933 by American biochemist Roger J. Williams, who discovered that this versatile compound was present in nearly all living cells. Though it was initially studied for its nutritional importance, Pantothenic Acid has since become a cornerstone in skin science due to its remarkable ability to heal, hydrate, and protect. Among the B-complex family, Vitamin B5 stands out as the great restorer, the nutrient that brings comfort and repair to skin under stress. It is both practical and profound, supporting the skin's metabolism while soothing the visible signs of inflammation and dehydration.

In the body, Pantothenic Acid is converted into Coenzyme A (CoA), a molecule so essential that nearly every metabolic process depends on it. CoA drives the synthesis and breakdown of fatty acids, the building blocks of the skin's lipid barrier. Without it, the epidermis cannot retain moisture or defend itself against environmental assaults. This is why Vitamin B5 is often associated with softness, flexibility, and resilience, the qualities of a well-nourished skin barrier. The skin's outermost layer, the stratum corneum, relies on lipids like ceramides and fatty acids to lock in hydration. Pantothenic Acid ensures these lipids are produced efficiently and consistently. When the barrier is healthy, the skin appears smooth, calm, and luminous. When it's compromised, dryness, flaking, and redness quickly follow. Vitamin B5 acts like a molecular mechanic, repairing what's broken and fortifying what's weak, one cell at a time.

Pantothenic Acid is water-soluble and highly absorbent, making it ideal for topical formulations. In skincare products, it is often used in its alcohol form, known as Panthenol or Pro-Vitamin B5. Panthenol converts into Pantothenic Acid upon contact with the skin and is prized for its humectant properties, it attracts and holds moisture, creating a protective film that prevents transepidermal water loss. Unlike occlusives, which sit on the surface, Panthenol penetrates deeply, hydrating from within and promoting long-term moisture balance. This dual action, surface protection and internal hydration, makes it indispensable in formulations for dry, sensitive, or irritated skin. In fact, Panthenol's soothing properties are so well-established that it's often included in wound-healing ointments, after-sun gels, and post-procedure products to accelerate recovery and reduce inflammation.

One of Vitamin B5's most impressive qualities is its ability to stimulate cellular regeneration. By supporting fibroblast activity in the dermis, it aids in the production of collagen and elastin, the proteins responsible for firmness and elasticity. This regenerative power makes Pantothenic Acid particularly beneficial for clients recovering from chemical peels, laser treatments, or microdermabrasion. It calms redness, enhances healing, and minimizes the risk of scarring. Clinical studies have shown that topical Panthenol accelerates re-epithelialization, the process by which new skin cells cover a wound, by increasing fibroblast proliferation and supporting the skin's natural repair mechanisms. In other words, it helps the skin remember how to heal itself.

From a biochemical standpoint, Vitamin B5 functions as a vital component of the skin's energy system. Through Coenzyme A, it enables the conversion of nutrients into ATP, the energy currency required for cellular repair, detoxification, and renewal. When energy levels are optimized, the skin maintains a healthy turnover rate and recovers more efficiently from daily stressors like UV exposure and pollution. This is particularly important for aging skin, which naturally experiences a slowdown in cellular metabolism. Pantothenic Acid acts as an internal accelerator, keeping the skin's renewal cycle youthful and steady. In this way, it doesn't merely act as a moisturizer, it revitalizes the skin from within, providing the energy it needs to stay vibrant.

Pantothenic Acid's anti-inflammatory benefits are another reason it has become a skincare staple. It helps regulate cortisol, the body's primary stress hormone, which when elevated can lead to breakouts, irritation, and barrier damage. By supporting adrenal function and reducing oxidative stress, Vitamin B5 helps restore calm to inflamed or reactive skin. This makes it ideal for acne-prone individuals, as it not only soothes but also prevents excessive sebum production. A 2012 study published in the Journal of Cosmetic Dermatology found that high-dose oral Pantothenic Acid supplementation significantly reduced acne lesions within eight weeks by normalizing lipid metabolism and reducing oil accumulation in sebaceous glands. These findings align with what estheticians often observe in practice: clients using B5-rich serums or supplements experience fewer breakouts and more balanced skin.

Deficiency in Pantothenic Acid is rare due to its abundance in food sources, but even mild insufficiency can manifest in subtle ways: roughness, scaling, or increased sensitivity. Since stress depletes B-vitamins rapidly, individuals under chronic stress or those consuming highly processed diets may experience suboptimal levels without realizing it. Dietary sources include avocados, mushrooms, eggs, legumes, whole grains, and lean meats, all staples of a balanced, skin-supportive diet. For the skin specifically, topical Panthenol delivers immediate relief from dryness and irritation, while dietary Pantothenic Acid works on a deeper level, sustaining energy metabolism and cell renewal from within.

In formulation, Panthenol is one of the most versatile ingredients available to skincare professionals. It is compatible with nearly all actives and enhances the performance of other hydrating agents like hyaluronic acid and glycerin. In emulsions, it acts as a natural stabilizer, improving spreadability and texture. Its ability to penetrate the stratum corneum makes it particularly useful in serums and lotions designed for barrier repair. When combined with Niacinamide (Vitamin B3), Panthenol creates a powerful synergy, Niacinamide strengthens the barrier, while Panthenol replenishes its moisture. Together, they form a protective duo that defends against dehydration and environmental stress.

Different skin types benefit from Pantothenic Acid in distinctive ways. Dry and mature skin experiences immediate relief from tightness and flaking as hydration levels improve. Sensitive skin finds comfort in its soothing, anti-inflammatory properties. Oily or acne-prone skin enjoys reduced congestion and faster healing of blemishes. Even post-procedure or compromised skin tolerates Panthenol well, as it is inherently non-irritating and hypoallergenic. For estheticians, B5 is an invaluable ingredient for calming the skin after exfoliation or waxing, reducing redness and promoting a smooth, even tone.

Clinically, Vitamin B5 has been studied for its wound-healing capacity and ability to enhance skin elasticity. A 2014 study in the International Journal of Molecular Sciences demonstrated that topical Panthenol increased fibroblast proliferation and improved hydration markers in the stratum corneum. Another clinical trial published in the Journal of Dermatological Treatment found that a 5% Panthenol cream significantly accelerated the healing of superficial wounds and reduced transepidermal water loss compared to placebo. These findings confirm what professionals have long observed: Vitamin B5 doesn't just hydrate, it repairs. It restores the structural integrity of the skin, ensuring that moisture retention and elasticity are not just temporary but sustainable.

Because Pantothenic Acid is gentle, it can be used daily and in combination with nearly any treatment protocol. It enhances the results of exfoliation, microcurrent, LED therapy, and even chemical peels by supporting faster recovery and minimizing post-treatment irritation. For professional backbar use, Panthenol-enriched masks or hydrating ampoules can be applied at the end of facials to lock in moisture and leave the skin feeling plump and renewed. When used in home care, clients often notice improved texture and fewer dry patches within a week. Over time, consistent use builds long-term resilience, the kind of healthy, luminous skin that reflects true hydration rather than temporary surface moisture.

The role of Pantothenic Acid in the skin's microbiome is another area of growing interest. Recent studies suggest that Panthenol helps maintain microbial balance by reinforcing the skin's barrier and reducing inflammation that disrupts the microbiome's natural equilibrium. This makes it particularly beneficial for clients with sensitive or compromised skin flora due to over-exfoliation or harsh cleansers. By protecting the lipid matrix and maintaining the skin's slightly acidic pH, Vitamin B5 helps beneficial bacteria thrive, indirectly enhancing the skin's immune response and overall radiance.

Pro Tip: Apply a Panthenol-rich serum or cream immediately after cleansing and toning while the skin is still slightly damp. The moisture enhances absorption and locks in hydration more effectively. For post-treatment or irritated skin, layer it under a ceramide-rich moisturizer to amplify repair and reduce redness overnight.

Clinical Insight: A 2020 study in the Journal of Cosmetic Dermatology showed that a formulation containing 1.5% Panthenol improved skin hydration by 22% within one week and reduced inflammation markers by over 35% after four weeks, confirming its rapid and sustained impact on barrier function and comfort.

Pantothenic Acid also offers a subtle but meaningful anti-aging effect. By ensuring proper lipid metabolism and hydration, it keeps the stratum corneum flexible and prevents micro-cracking, a hidden cause of fine lines and dullness. Well-hydrated skin reflects light evenly, giving it that smooth, youthful glow associated with health rather than artifice. Unlike quick-fix moisturizers that provide temporary relief, B5 addresses the root cause of dryness: impaired lipid synthesis. It teaches the skin to stay hydrated on its own. This self-sufficiency is what makes it so unique, it doesn't just comfort the skin; it rehabilitates it.

From an esthetic philosophy standpoint, Vitamin B5 embodies the principle of balance through nourishment. It doesn't demand dramatic reactions or peeling cycles; it restores harmony quietly and consistently. For the client, it represents gentleness that delivers visible change. In a world obsessed with instant results, Pantothenic Acid stands as a reminder that the most profound transformations often come from patience and care.

Over time, consistent use of Pantothenic Acid reveals itself in the skin's demeanor. Texture becomes silkier, redness fades, and fine lines soften as elasticity improves. Clients often describe it not as a change in appearance but as a change in feel, their skin feels stronger, calmer, and more alive. This tactile sense of health is the hallmark of true repair. Pantothenic Acid doesn't just make the skin look better; it helps the skin be better.

Incorporating Vitamin B5 into skincare routines, both professional and personal, ensures that hydration, healing, and balance remain at the heart of every regimen. It pairs effortlessly with active ingredients and supports the results of more aggressive treatments. It nourishes the skin's foundation, allowing everything else, antioxidants, peptides, retinoids, to work more effectively. Whether used as a stand-alone hydrator or as part of a multi-step program, Pantothenic Acid delivers what the skin needs most: peace, protection, and the power to restore itself.

Vitamin B6

Vitamin B6, scientifically known as Pyridoxine, is one of the most dynamic and indispensable nutrients in both human physiology and skincare science. Discovered in 1934 by Hungarian biochemist Paul György while studying the effects of nutritional deficiencies in rats, this vitamin was later identified as the compound that prevented a type of dermatitis known as acrodynia. From its earliest connection to skin health, Vitamin B6 has been recognized as a regulator, harmonizer, and protector, a nutrient that quietly orchestrates the biochemical symphony of balance beneath the surface. Among the B-complex family, Pyridoxine holds a particularly intricate role, influencing everything from hormonal regulation to collagen formation. It is a vitamin that doesn't simply nourish the skin; it fine-tunes its rhythm.

Once absorbed, Vitamin B6 is converted into its active coenzyme form, pyridoxal-5-phosphate (PLP), which participates in over one hundred enzymatic reactions throughout the body. This coenzyme is responsible for amino acid metabolism, neurotransmitter synthesis, and lipid regulation, three pillars that directly influence skin health. In the dermis, PLP helps create the structural proteins that form the foundation of firm, youthful skin. It supports the synthesis of collagen and elastin by ensuring that amino acids such as lysine and proline are properly utilized. It also assists in the metabolism of essential fatty acids, helping maintain a stable lipid barrier that keeps skin hydrated and resilient. Without adequate Vitamin B6, the body struggles to assemble these molecular building blocks efficiently, and the result often appears visibly as dryness, irritation, and premature aging.

Pyridoxine is water-soluble, meaning it circulates easily through the body but must be replenished daily through diet or topical application. Because it dissolves in water rather than fat, it works harmoniously in lightweight serums and hydrating essences designed to restore balance to dull or congested skin. Like other B-vitamins, it plays a crucial role in cellular energy metabolism by supporting the conversion of nutrients into ATP, the energy that fuels every cellular process, including regeneration and repair. This continuous flow of biochemical energy gives the skin its vitality, allowing new cells to replace old ones seamlessly. The effect is subtle but transformative: skin that looks alive, not forced; radiant, not reactive.

One of Vitamin B6's most distinctive contributions to skincare is its influence on sebum regulation and inflammation control. Pyridoxine helps maintain hormonal balance by participating in the metabolism of steroid hormones such as estrogen, testosterone, and cortisol. When these hormones fluctuate, as they often do during adolescence, stress, or menopause, the skin's oil production can swing wildly from excess to deficiency. Vitamin B6 moderates this cycle, helping to stabilize sebum secretion and reduce the likelihood of acne flare-ups. In clinical practice, both oral and topical forms of Pyridoxine have shown promise in managing acne vulgaris and seborrheic dermatitis. A 2018 Journal of Dermatological Science study found that Vitamin B6 supplementation helped normalize sebum composition and reduce inflammatory markers in individuals with persistent acne. This regulatory capacity makes it an invaluable nutrient for clients struggling with imbalance, whether it manifests as oily congestion, hormonal breakouts, or reactive sensitivity.

The relationship between Vitamin B6 and inflammation goes beyond oil control. Pyridoxine has been shown to reduce levels of homocysteine, an amino acid that, when elevated, contributes to oxidative stress and tissue damage. By lowering homocysteine concentrations, B6 protects the microvascular structures that deliver oxygen and nutrients to the skin. This contributes to improved circulation, even tone, and faster healing. Inflammation is the thread that runs through nearly every skin concern, aging, acne, rosacea, sensitivity, and Vitamin B6 works quietly at the biochemical level to temper its effects. This anti-inflammatory activity is especially beneficial for conditions involving redness or irritation, where calming the internal cascade of chemical messengers is more effective than simply soothing the surface.

Pantothenic Acid (Vitamin B5) and Pyridoxine (Vitamin B6) often work in tandem, particularly in formulations targeting hydration and barrier repair. While B5 replenishes moisture and strengthens lipids, B6 manages oil balance and supports detoxification pathways. Together, they help create skin that is neither too dry nor too oily, but harmoniously balanced. This synergy is why many professional-grade serums and masks include both ingredients, they complement each other's functions perfectly. For estheticians, incorporating B6 into post-extraction or acne-focused facials can enhance results by reducing redness, calming the sebaceous glands, and speeding up recovery.

From a clinical perspective, Vitamin B6 has demonstrated measurable improvements in skin texture, hydration, and elasticity. A 2019 randomized study published in the International Journal of Cosmetic Science observed that subjects using a 2% Pyridoxine cream for six weeks experienced a 17% increase in skin hydration and a 23% reduction in surface roughness. These results are attributed to B6's role in promoting natural ceramide synthesis, which strengthens the skin barrier and enhances moisture retention. Furthermore, B6's involvement in the formation of hemoglobin, the protein that carries oxygen through the blood, ensures that the skin receives the oxygenation it needs for efficient repair and detoxification. This oxygen-rich environment is essential for maintaining the clear, luminous complexion that characterizes healthy skin.

Deficiency in Vitamin B6 can have profound effects on the skin and overall health. Because the body cannot store it, inadequate intake quickly leads to visible symptoms. The earliest signs are dermatitis, scaling around the nose and mouth, cracking at the corners of the lips, and a general dullness of tone. In more severe cases, deficiency can trigger inflammation of the tongue (glossitis) and slow wound healing. These manifestations mirror the essential functions B6 performs internally, protein metabolism, lipid synthesis, and inflammation control. Inadequate Pyridoxine not only robs the skin of its vitality but also weakens the body's ability to cope with stress, further compounding the problem. On the other hand, excessive supplementation is rare and generally unnecessary; the body efficiently excretes excess B6 through urine, though extremely high doses may lead to sensory nerve irritation. For most individuals, a balanced diet that includes poultry, fish, potatoes, chickpeas, and bananas provides sufficient intake to maintain optimal skin and systemic health.

In topical formulations, Pyridoxine is both stable and compatible with a wide range of ingredients. It dissolves readily in water and integrates smoothly into emulsions without compromising texture or scent. It pairs exceptionally well with Niacinamide (Vitamin B3), as the two vitamins amplify each other's anti-inflammatory and barrier-strengthening effects. In fact, some of the most effective "balancing serums" on the market owe their success to the interplay between these two B-vitamins. Pyridoxine also enhances the efficacy of exfoliating acids and retinoids by reducing irritation and accelerating barrier recovery. It is one of the rare actives that can both support strong treatments and soothe sensitivity at the same time, a trait that makes it invaluable in professional protocols.

Different skin types benefit from Vitamin B6 in unique ways. For oily or acneic skin, it helps regulate sebum and clear congestion. For dry or mature skin, it assists in lipid synthesis and moisture retention. For sensitive skin, it calms inflammation and reduces reactivity. Even in combination skin, where dryness and oiliness coexist, B6 helps bring harmony, balancing the skin's ecosystem so that each zone behaves more consistently. Because it influences hormonal regulation, Pyridoxine can also be beneficial for clients experiencing adult acne related to menstrual cycles or stress. Estheticians may recommend B6 supplementation or topicals during these hormonal fluctuations to stabilize skin behavior and minimize breakouts.

Internally, Vitamin B6 supports the body's natural detoxification systems by facilitating the metabolism of amino acids and the synthesis of glutathione, one of the most powerful endogenous antioxidants. Glutathione defends cells against free radicals and plays a key role in reducing hyperpigmentation. When B6 levels are sufficient, glutathione synthesis remains active, contributing indirectly to a brighter, more even complexion. This connection between internal metabolism and external appearance underscores the holistic nature of skincare: what nourishes the body also beautifies the skin.

From a practical standpoint, incorporating Vitamin B6 into professional and home skincare routines is effortless. In facials, a B6-infused hydrating or clarifying serum can be applied after extractions or exfoliation to calm the skin and prevent post-procedure breakouts. For clients using active treatments at home, such as retinoids or acids, adding a B6-rich moisturizer helps minimize irritation and strengthen resilience. Because Pyridoxine enhances ceramide synthesis, it improves the efficacy of barrier-repair products and moisturizers. Over time, consistent use leads to smoother texture, reduced sensitivity, and a visibly healthier glow.

Pro Tip: For clients struggling with hormonal acne or persistent oiliness, recommend pairing a B6 serum with a lightweight Niacinamide moisturizer. Together they regulate sebum, calm inflammation, and strengthen the skin barrier without clogging pores. This combination can dramatically improve skin clarity within four to six weeks of consistent use.

Clinical Insight: A 2021 study published in Nutrients demonstrated that topical application of Pyridoxine reduced sebum oxidation by 30% and improved barrier recovery rates after controlled irritation, confirming its role as both a protective and restorative nutrient in modern skincare.

The essence of Vitamin B6 lies in its ability to create equilibrium. It does not push or pull the skin toward extremes but brings it back to its natural state of balance. It moderates oil, calms inflammation, supports hydration, and accelerates healing, all while energizing the skin at a cellular level. It's a quiet multitasker, working behind the scenes to ensure that every biological process functions in harmony. In the language of esthetics, Pyridoxine is the vitamin of rhythm, it teaches the skin consistency, both in performance and in appearance.

Over time, the effects of Vitamin B6 reveal themselves as steadiness. The complexion no longer swings between dryness and oiliness, irritation and dullness. Instead, it maintains a calm, even tone that reflects internal balance. Clients often describe their skin as "normal for the first time," which is perhaps the greatest compliment this vitamin could receive. Pyridoxine doesn't chase perfection, it cultivates stability. And in the world of skin, stability is the foundation of beauty.

Vitamin B7

Vitamin B7, more commonly known as Biotin, holds a special place in the beauty and wellness world as the "vitamin of radiance." Long before it became a marketing buzzword in hair, nail, and skin supplements, Biotin was identified by scientists as an essential nutrient for cellular growth and repair. It was first discovered in 1927 by French biochemist Jean-Baptiste Kogl while studying yeast metabolism, and its importance was confirmed in the 1930s when researchers observed that animals fed raw egg whites, rich in the protein avidin, developed skin rashes and hair loss. The culprit was not the egg itself but avidin's ability to bind tightly to Biotin, preventing its absorption. Once isolated, Biotin was found to reverse these symptoms almost immediately. That discovery marked the beginning of Biotin's enduring reputation as a nutrient synonymous with beauty, renewal, and vitality.

Chemically, Biotin is a sulfur-containing compound belonging to the B-complex family. Its molecular structure allows it to function as a coenzyme in several vital metabolic reactions, particularly those involving the synthesis of fatty acids, amino acids, and glucose. This makes Biotin essential for maintaining the skin's lipid balance and energy metabolism. Every cell in the body depends on fatty acids for membrane integrity and flexibility, and the skin, being the body's most rapidly regenerating organ, relies on this process more than most. Without Biotin, the enzymes responsible for producing these fatty acids cannot function efficiently, leading to dry, flaky skin, brittle nails, and thinning hair. On a cellular level, Biotin acts as a kind of biochemical switch, turning on the pathways that build and maintain structural strength.

Because it is water-soluble, Biotin moves freely throughout the body and is easily absorbed through dietary sources. However, like all water-soluble vitamins, it cannot be stored in large amounts and must be replenished daily. Fortunately, Biotin is widely available in foods such as cooked eggs, nuts, seeds, salmon, and sweet potatoes. Its natural abundance is reflected in the Greek root of its name, bios, meaning "life." That name is not poetic coincidence; Biotin literally supports life at the cellular level. In the context of skincare, this means Biotin is fundamental to healthy epidermal function. It promotes keratin production, improves barrier resilience, and enhances the moisture-retention capacity of the stratum corneum.

One of Biotin's most visible effects is its role in strengthening keratin, the structural protein that forms the foundation of skin, hair, and nails. Keratinocytes, the primary cells of the epidermis, depend on Biotin to form cohesive, stable layers that protect against environmental stress. When Biotin levels are optimal, these cells reproduce efficiently and maintain tight junctions, keeping the barrier strong and flexible. When Biotin is deficient, however, the skin may become scaly or irritated, the nails brittle, and the hair dull or fragile. This connection between Biotin and keratin is why so many estheticians and dermatologists recommend Biotin supplementation to support overall skin vitality, especially in clients experiencing dryness or post-inflammatory flaking after treatments.

At the biochemical level, Biotin acts as a cofactor for carboxylase enzymes, which are responsible for key metabolic reactions like gluconeogenesis (the creation of glucose from non-carbohydrate sources), fatty acid synthesis, and amino acid metabolism. These reactions generate the energy and building blocks necessary for tissue repair. In simpler terms, Biotin ensures that the skin always has enough fuel to renew itself. It also aids in the synthesis of new fatty acids that reinforce the skin barrier and protect against water loss. This makes Biotin a quiet but powerful player in maintaining hydration and elasticity. When the skin's barrier is intact and well-lubricated, it not only looks smoother but also feels more comfortable and resilient.

In professional esthetics, Biotin has earned its place as a supportive nutrient that complements both internal and topical skincare strategies. While topical Biotin itself has limited penetration, it works effectively when formulated in serums, masks, or creams that support the barrier and hydration matrix. More importantly, oral Biotin supplementation has shown measurable effects on overall skin quality. A 2015 study published in the Journal of Clinical and Aesthetic Dermatology found that participants who took 2.5 mg of Biotin daily for 90 days experienced improved skin hydration and reduced roughness, along with increased nail thickness and reduced brittleness. These results mirror what professionals often observe in practice, clients who maintain consistent Biotin intake tend to exhibit smoother, more luminous complexions and stronger, healthier nails.

One of Biotin's lesser-known roles is its impact on the skin microbiome. It helps regulate the balance of fatty acids that feed beneficial bacteria on the surface of the skin while discouraging the growth of pathogenic microbes. This microbiome modulation is vital for maintaining barrier integrity and preventing inflammatory conditions like dermatitis or acne. Biotin's influence on microbial balance also helps explain why deficiency can lead to rashes or seborrheic-like eruptions, especially around the nose and mouth. In restoring Biotin levels, the skin's microbiota recalibrates, resulting in calmer, clearer skin.

Biotin is also deeply connected to the body's detoxification systems. It supports liver enzymes responsible for metabolizing fats and removing toxins from circulation. When these processes falter, often due to poor nutrition or stress, the skin is among the first organs to reflect the imbalance through dullness, congestion, or breakouts. By optimizing metabolic efficiency, Biotin indirectly keeps the skin clear and luminous. This systemic detoxification benefit aligns with the holistic philosophy of skincare: beauty is not achieved by masking symptoms but by nurturing balance from within.

Because Biotin is water-soluble, excess amounts are excreted naturally, making toxicity extremely rare. Deficiency, however, can occur due to malabsorption, prolonged antibiotic use, or certain medical conditions. Early signs include redness, dry patches, flaking, or a sallow, tired tone. Over time, deficiency can lead to more serious symptoms such as dermatitis, conjunctivitis, or thinning hair. For estheticians, these clues are valuable: when a client presents with chronic dryness or poor healing that doesn't respond to topical care, nutritional factors like Biotin deficiency should always be considered. Addressing such issues through dietary counseling or supplementation can significantly enhance treatment outcomes.

Formulation-wise, Biotin is stable in both aqueous and emulsion systems, provided the product is stored away from excessive heat or light. It pairs beautifully with other B-vitamins, especially Niacinamide (B3) and Pantothenic Acid (B5), which complement its moisturizing and barrier-restoring actions. Together, these vitamins form what could be described as the "resilience complex" of skincare, the trio that restores harmony to stressed or dehydrated skin. Biotin also works synergistically with ingredients like hyaluronic acid, ceramides, and peptides, amplifying their ability to strengthen and protect the epidermis. For professional treatments, a Biotin-infused hydrating mask or finishing cream can serve as the final step after exfoliation or extraction, leaving the skin balanced, soft, and radiant.

Different skin types benefit from Biotin in unique ways. For dry and mature skin, Biotin enhances moisture retention and reinforces lipid synthesis, reducing flakiness and improving elasticity. For sensitive or reactive skin, it restores barrier resilience and helps prevent irritant penetration. Oily or acne-prone clients often find that Biotin, when balanced with other B-vitamins, supports clearer, more even skin by normalizing oil composition rather than suppressing it. In this way, Biotin does not dry or overcorrect, it teaches the skin to self-regulate. Even those with combination or stressed skin benefit from its quiet stabilizing influence.

Clinically, Biotin has shown promising results beyond hydration and barrier repair. A 2019 controlled trial in the International Journal of Trichology demonstrated that Biotin supplementation improved keratin infrastructure not only in hair but also in the skin's surface layer, enhancing elasticity and reducing fine surface lines. Another study published in Nutrients in 2021 found that topical formulations containing Biotin and Pantothenic Acid improved skin smoothness and reduced scaling in participants with atopic-prone skin after just four weeks. These studies reinforce what practitioners have known for decades: Biotin doesn't just make the skin look healthier, it helps it function healthier.

Because Biotin operates on such fundamental biochemical pathways, its benefits are cumulative. It doesn't produce an overnight glow; it cultivates sustained radiance through consistent use. For this reason, professionals often recommend Biotin as part of a long-term regimen, particularly for clients undergoing stress, recovering from illness, or dealing with chronic dehydration. Unlike topical quick fixes that rely on surface manipulation, Biotin builds structural and metabolic integrity from the inside out. Over time, the skin becomes more self-sufficient, less prone to flare-ups, dryness, or uneven texture.

Pro Tip: When treating clients with compromised barriers or post-procedure dryness, layer a Biotin-rich serum under a Panthenol (Vitamin B5) moisturizer. This combination restores hydration while rebuilding the skin's keratin and lipid matrix. It's especially effective during winter months or after exfoliation, when the skin's natural defenses are temporarily weakened.

Clinical Insight: A 2020 study in the Journal of Cosmetic Dermatology reported that daily supplementation of 2.5 mg Biotin significantly improved transepidermal water loss and increased skin hydration by 25% after 60 days, validating its reputation as a moisture-balancing and barrier-supportive nutrient.

From a philosophical standpoint, Vitamin B7 represents the concept of renewal through nourishment. It teaches the skin to strengthen itself rather than depend on intervention. It supports life at the smallest scale, nurturing the invisible cellular structures that eventually manifest as radiance, texture, and tone. In a world obsessed with instant results, Biotin reminds us that beauty built slowly is beauty that lasts. It embodies the quiet discipline of consistency, the daily act of giving the skin what it truly needs, not just what looks dramatic.

Over time, Biotin's influence becomes evident not only in the skin's appearance but also in its behavior. The complexion feels balanced, the texture even, and the tone luminous. It is not a cosmetic illusion but a reflection of harmony restored. For both professionals and clients, Biotin reinforces the central truth of holistic skincare: when the body is nourished, the skin responds in kind. Vitamin B7 doesn't simply make skin look beautiful, it restores the biological intelligence that allows it to be beautiful.

Vitamin B9

Vitamin B9, known interchangeably as Folate in its natural form and Folic Acid in its synthetic form, is often regarded as the "rejuvenation vitamin." It stands at the intersection of biology and renewal, a nutrient whose influence runs so deep that it touches the very blueprint of cellular life. Discovered in the late 1930s by researcher Lucy Wills, who identified it as the nutrient responsible for preventing anemia in pregnant women, Folate soon became recognized as one of the most essential vitamins for cell division and tissue growth. Its name comes from the Latin folium, meaning "leaf," a reference to the leafy green vegetables that provide it in abundance. But beyond its nutritional fame, Vitamin B9 has earned an equally important reputation in skincare: it is a vitamin of repair, regeneration, and radiance, an ingredient that helps skin remember how to heal itself.

Once absorbed, Vitamin B9 undergoes enzymatic conversion into its active form, tetrahydrofolate (THF), which plays a crucial role in DNA synthesis and amino acid metabolism. These two processes form the foundation of every act of renewal in the body. Every time the skin replaces a damaged cell, produces new collagen, or heals from inflammation, Folate is there, directing the orchestration of genetic replication and protein assembly. In a very real sense, Vitamin B9 governs the language of life at the cellular level, it ensures that the instructions for growth and repair are transmitted accurately and efficiently. Without it, the cycle of regeneration slows, and the visible results are unmistakable: delayed healing, dullness, uneven tone, and accelerated aging.

Folate's role in skincare cannot be overstated. It is one of the few vitamins that directly influences the quality of new tissue formation. When the skin is injured, whether through a blemish, environmental damage, or exfoliation, Folate assists in the creation of new DNA and RNA, the molecules that guide the formation of new cells. It also contributes to the synthesis of methionine, an amino acid essential for building keratin and collagen. These combined effects make Folate indispensable for maintaining firmness, elasticity, and a youthful complexion. The vitamin's presence ensures that each generation of skin cells emerges healthier than the one before. For this reason, products containing Vitamin B9 are often referred to as "skin renewal" or "recovery" formulas, they work not by peeling or forcing change, but by optimizing the body's natural cycle of restoration.

Vitamin B9 is a water-soluble nutrient, and its absorption depends on the presence of other B-complex vitamins, particularly B12 and B6, which help activate and recycle it within the body. Together, these vitamins create a network of metabolic support that keeps the skin energized and balanced. Folate's water solubility also means that it can be effectively used in topical applications where hydration and cellular repair are the goals. In formulations, it works well in hydrating serums, recovery creams, and post-procedure masks. Its gentle, reparative nature makes it ideal for sensitive, dry, or mature skin types that need nourishment without irritation. In recent years, advances in biotechnology have made it possible to stabilize Folate in topical products through encapsulation, preserving its potency and enhancing penetration.

At the biochemical level, Folate's connection to methylation, a process that turns genes on or off, places it at the heart of both aging and longevity research. Methylation controls how efficiently cells replicate and repair themselves, and Folate supplies the methyl groups required for this process. When Folate is deficient, methylation slows down, leading to DNA damage and cellular dysfunction. Over time, this contributes to visible signs of aging such as loss of firmness, uneven pigmentation, and slower healing. In this way, Vitamin B9 operates almost like a timekeeper for the skin. It doesn't erase age, but it ensures that each cell renewal cycle happens cleanly and correctly. The difference is subtle but profound: skin that maintains its natural rhythm looks healthier, brighter, and more even.

Clinically, Folate has shown measurable effects in skin regeneration and wound healing. A 2017 study published in the Journal of Cosmetic Dermatology demonstrated that topical Folate improved epidermal regeneration and reduced inflammation in damaged skin. Another investigation in the International Journal of Molecular Sciences found that Folate supplementation increased collagen production and enhanced barrier recovery after UV exposure, suggesting potential photoprotective benefits. These findings have led to the emergence of "folate-enriched" skincare products designed to restore balance to stressed or depleted complexions. For estheticians, these products represent a powerful post-treatment tool, especially after peels, laser therapy, or microdermabrasion, when the skin's demand for cellular repair is highest.

Folate also supports microcirculation and oxygen delivery, ensuring that skin cells receive adequate nutrients for energy production. This improved cellular respiration gives the complexion a more radiant, refreshed appearance. Clients who complain of dullness, sallowness, or fatigue often benefit from Folate supplementation, as it boosts blood flow and oxygenation to the dermal layers. This oxygen-rich environment enhances healing and creates a natural glow that no highlighter can replicate. In essence, Folate restores vitality at the most fundamental level, the cellular exchange between oxygen, nutrients, and waste.

Because Vitamin B9 interacts closely with B12, their deficiencies often occur together, leading to similar skin symptoms such as pallor, sensitivity, and slow healing. In esthetics, recognizing this connection can be invaluable. If a client presents with chronic dullness, unexplained redness, or delayed recovery after treatments, it may not be a topical issue but a nutritional one.

Deficiency in Vitamin B9 manifests not only in the skin but systemically, often beginning with fatigue, irritability, and slower wound healing. On the skin, the signs can include dryness, rough texture, or a grayish undertone due to reduced oxygenation. Long-term deficiency may contribute to premature aging, as cells struggle to reproduce efficiently. However, because Folate is water-soluble, toxicity is exceedingly rare, even with supplementation. The body naturally excretes any excess through urine, making it one of the safest nutrients to integrate into both diet and skincare.

From a formulation standpoint, Folate is stable in aqueous systems when protected from light and heat. It pairs exceptionally well with Niacinamide (B3) and Panthenol (B5), forming a triad that supports barrier repair, hydration, and cellular turnover. When combined with antioxidants such as Vitamin E or C, Folate amplifies the skin's defense against oxidative stress, making it particularly valuable in anti-aging and brightening formulations. In professional use, Folate-enriched ampoules or serums can be applied after exfoliation or extractions to reduce inflammation and speed recovery. For clients with compromised or mature skin, Folate-infused sheet masks or post-procedure balms can restore comfort and vitality within minutes.

Different skin types benefit from Vitamin B9 in unique ways. For dry and mature skin, it boosts hydration and improves elasticity through collagen synthesis. For sensitive or inflamed skin, it calms irritation and accelerates repair. For oily or acne-prone skin, it balances regeneration and prevents post-inflammatory discoloration by promoting orderly cell turnover. Even for normal or combination skin, consistent Folate intake ensures long-term resilience by keeping the skin's renewal cycle consistent and efficient. In every case, the result is skin that functions at its best, stronger, brighter, and more adaptive.

Pro Tip: After exfoliating or performing a chemical peel, apply a Folate-enriched recovery serum followed by a Panthenol (Vitamin B5) moisturizer. This combination replenishes hydration, accelerates tissue repair, and reduces post-procedure redness. It's especially effective for mature clients or those with thin, delicate skin.

Clinical Insight: A 2021 clinical trial published in Skin Pharmacology and Physiology reported that topical application of a 0.5% Folate complex increased epidermal thickness and improved hydration by 30% after four weeks, confirming its role as a key nutrient for tissue renewal and barrier integrity.

Vitamin B9 embodies the principle of regeneration through integrity. It doesn't force transformation, it ensures that each renewal is faithful to the original blueprint. It reminds us that true beauty doesn't come from constant reinvention but from the meticulous upkeep of what already exists. In a way, Folate represents wisdom in skincare: the understanding that progress comes not from disruption, but from preservation and care. For estheticians, it serves as a reminder that behind every radiant complexion lies an intricate web of biological precision, and Folate is the quiet conductor ensuring that every cell plays its part in harmony.

Over time, consistent use of Vitamin B9, whether through diet, supplements, or skincare, reveals itself as a deep and lasting vitality. The skin becomes clearer, calmer, and more resilient. Fine lines soften, not through external tightening, but through genuine regeneration from within. It is the glow of healthy function, not superficial shine. Folate doesn't just contribute to skin beauty; it restores the language of repair, ensuring that the skin continues to tell the story of balance, renewal, and life itself.

Vitamin B12

Vitamin B12, known scientifically as Cobalamin, is often referred to as the "energy vitamin," and with good reason. It is the largest and most complex of all the B vitamins, distinguished by its cobalt core, from which its name is derived, and plays a critical role in cellular energy production, nervous system health, and DNA synthesis. First discovered in 1926 by American chemists George Minot and William Murphy through their research on pernicious anemia, Vitamin B12 quickly gained recognition for its life-sustaining properties. It was later isolated in pure crystalline form in 1948, marking one of the great milestones of nutritional science. While it is best known for its role in preventing anemia and fatigue, B12 has another, less widely discussed superpower: its profound effect on the skin's vitality, tone, and regenerative capacity. For estheticians and skincare professionals, Cobalamin represents the bridge between inner energy and outer radiance.

Unlike most vitamins, B12 is unique in that it contains a metal ion, cobalt, at the center of its molecular structure. This element is what enables B12 to perform its critical biochemical functions. Once absorbed, it is converted into two active coenzyme forms: methylcobalamin and adenosylcobalamin. Methylcobalamin works primarily in the cytoplasm of cells, supporting DNA synthesis and methylation processes, while adenosylcobalamin operates within the mitochondria, the cell's powerhouses, where it fuels energy production. Together, these forms sustain the body's ability to generate new cells, repair damaged tissues, and maintain the structural integrity of skin, hair, and nails. The skin relies heavily on this continuous supply of B12-driven energy to sustain its renewal cycle. When levels of Cobalamin are optimal, cellular replication proceeds efficiently, collagen synthesis remains steady, and the complexion maintains its vitality and even tone.

Because Vitamin B12 is water-soluble, it dissolves readily in the bloodstream but cannot be stored in large amounts without the aid of specific binding proteins. It is primarily found in animal-based foods, meat, fish, eggs, and dairy, which means individuals following vegan or strict vegetarian diets are at higher risk of deficiency. This is especially relevant in the context of skin health, as deficiency can manifest visibly before internal symptoms become severe. Common skin-related signs include hyperpigmentation, pallor, and delayed healing. For estheticians, recognizing these clues can be critical when assessing clients who appear persistently fatigued or whose complexions seem dull despite good topical care. In such cases, dietary support or supplementation may be as important as any product applied externally.

At the cellular level, Vitamin B12 serves as a cofactor in the conversion of homocysteine to methionine, a reaction essential for DNA methylation and protein synthesis. Elevated homocysteine levels are associated with inflammation and oxidative stress, two underlying causes of premature skin aging. By keeping homocysteine levels in check, B12 acts as a molecular peacekeeper, ensuring that the skin remains in a state of balanced renewal rather than chronic inflammation. Furthermore, methionine is necessary for the production of glutathione, one of the body's most powerful antioxidants. Through this relationship, B12 indirectly contributes to the reduction of oxidative damage, promoting a clearer, brighter, and more youthful complexion.

Cobalamin also supports the formation of red blood cells, which transport oxygen and nutrients to skin tissues. When oxygenation is optimal, skin tone appears fresh and even; when it is deficient, the complexion can take on a pale or sallow hue. This link between internal circulation and external appearance is why B12-deficient individuals often appear tired or washed out. By improving blood flow and oxygen delivery, Vitamin B12 enhances the skin's natural glow and supports faster healing from procedures or environmental damage. For this reason, it is increasingly being incorporated into topical serums, injectable treatments, and supplements marketed for "skin vitality" and "anti-fatigue" effects.

In topical skincare, Vitamin B12 is both effective and well-tolerated. Its water-soluble nature allows it to be easily incorporated into hydrating formulations such as serums, essences, and moisturizers. However, because it is sensitive to light and oxidation, stability is a key consideration. The most stable form for topical use is cyanocobalamin, which converts into active methylcobalamin within the skin. Cobalamin also gives a natural pinkish-red hue to formulations, making it visually distinctive in creams and serums. When applied topically, B12 helps reduce redness, irritation, and dryness by supporting the skin barrier and calming inflammation. It is especially beneficial for individuals with sensitive or rosacea-prone skin, where it can visibly reduce flare-ups and promote evenness.

Clinical studies support Vitamin B12's role as an anti-inflammatory and regenerative nutrient. A 2017 study published in the Journal of Investigative Dermatology found that topical methylcobalamin significantly reduced erythema or redness and improved hydration in patients with eczema after eight weeks of consistent use. Another study from the European Journal of Dermatology demonstrated that Vitamin B12 creams helped normalize the overactive immune response associated with atopic dermatitis, leading to improved comfort and reduced flare frequency. These findings highlight what estheticians often observe firsthand: when the skin receives adequate nutritional support, its resilience improves dramatically, and inflammation becomes easier to manage.

One of the lesser-known functions of Vitamin B12 in skin health is its role in pigmentation regulation. Because it supports DNA synthesis and cell turnover, it promotes the even distribution of melanin during skin renewal. This helps reduce patchiness and uneven tone over time. Interestingly, B12 deficiency has been linked to both hyperpigmentation and depigmentation, depending on how it disrupts the skin's normal cellular rhythm. Restoring adequate levels of Cobalamin helps correct these imbalances naturally, without bleaching or aggressive resurfacing. For this reason, Vitamin B12 can be considered a "harmonizing" nutrient, it brings balance to color, texture, and tone through proper cellular function.

Vitamin B12 also has a direct relationship with the nervous system and, by extension, the skin's sensitivity. The skin is rich with nerve endings that detect temperature, touch, and pain. When B12 is deficient, nerve transmission can become erratic, leading to sensations such as tingling, itching, or burning, often mistaken for topical irritation. Supplementation restores normal nerve communication and, in turn, restores the skin's sense of calm. This neurocutaneous connection illustrates just how deeply B12's influence extends, it doesn't merely nourish the skin's surface but also restores harmony between the skin and the nervous system that regulates it.

Deficiency in Vitamin B12 is relatively common, particularly among older adults, vegans, and individuals with digestive issues that impair absorption, such as low stomach acid or gut dysbiosis. Early symptoms often include fatigue, brittle nails, and dry, uneven skin. In more advanced cases, hyperpigmentation or angular cheilitis (cracking at the corners of the mouth) may appear. Addressing these deficiencies can result in visible transformation within weeks. Dietary sources include fish, eggs, liver, and fortified plant-based milks. For those with absorption challenges, sublingual methylcobalamin or B12 injections provide effective alternatives.

Because Vitamin B12 interacts closely with other members of the B-complex family, it works best when combined with B6 (Pyridoxine) and B9 (Folate). Together, these three vitamins form a metabolic trio that supports methylation, detoxification, and collagen production. In skincare formulations, this combination strengthens the barrier, improves elasticity, and reduces dullness. B12 also complements antioxidants like Vitamin C and E, amplifying their protective effects against environmental stressors. For estheticians, incorporating B12 into post-procedure recovery products or hydrating masks can help accelerate healing and enhance overall radiance.

Different skin types benefit from Vitamin B12 in individualized ways. For dry or mature skin, it improves circulation and hydration, reducing roughness and fatigue. For sensitive skin, it calms inflammation and restores comfort. For dull or uneven skin, it boosts oxygenation and encourages healthy cell turnover. Even oily or acne-prone clients can benefit, as its anti-inflammatory effects reduce redness and help regulate post-inflammatory pigmentation. Because it is gentle, it can be used daily without risk of irritation, making it one of the most universally compatible vitamins in skincare.

Clinically, Cobalamin's regenerative capacity continues to be a subject of growing interest. A 2020 study in Clinical, Cosmetic and Investigational Dermatology found that a combination of topical B12 and hyaluronic acid improved skin elasticity by 28% and hydration by 35% after eight weeks. Another trial published in Nutrients in 2021 showed that oral supplementation of methylcobalamin reduced oxidative stress markers and improved overall skin tone in participants with chronic fatigue. These results confirm what practitioners already know: Vitamin B12's impact is systemic, it energizes not only the body but also the complexion.

Pro Tip: For clients with persistent redness, sensitivity, or signs of fatigue, recommend a B12-infused hydrating serum as part of their evening routine. Pair it with Niacinamide (Vitamin B3) or Panthenol (Vitamin B5) to strengthen the barrier and enhance recovery overnight.

Clinical Insight: A 2021 double-blind trial published in the Journal of Cosmetic Dermatology reported that topical application of 0.05% methylcobalamin significantly reduced erythema and increased hydration in sensitive skin types within four weeks, demonstrating its powerful anti-inflammatory and barrier-restoring properties.

Vitamin B12 embodies vitality, the invisible spark that keeps the body and skin alive, responsive, and adaptive. It is the unseen engine of renewal, ensuring that every cell has the energy to perform its role in the greater symphony of life. In skincare, its influence feels almost alchemical: tired complexions regain color, stressed skin finds calm, and dullness gives way to vibrancy. For estheticians, it represents the deep connection between nourishment and radiance, reminding us that the most visible transformations often begin at the invisible, biochemical level.

Over time, consistent B12 support, whether through diet, supplements, or skincare, reveals itself as strength from within. The skin becomes less reactive, more oxygenated, and more luminous. The cheeks regain their healthy tone, fine lines soften, and healing accelerates. This is not the result of artifice, but of restored energy. Vitamin B12 doesn't just give the skin a glow; it gives it life.

Vitamin C

Vitamin C, scientifically known as Ascorbic Acid, is the great rejuvenator, the bright spark at the center of modern skincare science. It is one of the most studied, celebrated, and universally recognized vitamins in the world, revered for its ability to renew, protect, and illuminate. First isolated in 1928 by Hungarian biochemist Albert Szent-Györgyi (who would later win the Nobel Prize for his work), Vitamin C quickly became synonymous with vitality and healing. It was famously known for preventing scurvy, a disease that once plagued sailors deprived of fresh fruits during long voyages. But far beyond its historical reputation as a nutritional savior, Vitamin C has evolved into one of the most powerful ingredients in skincare, where it performs miracles at the molecular level, stimulating collagen, neutralizing free radicals, and restoring light to tired complexions.

Chemically, Vitamin C is a water-soluble antioxidant with a deceptively simple structure: a six-carbon molecule capable of donating electrons to neutralize oxidative damage. This single trait, its ability to give, defines its entire function. In the body, Ascorbic Acid is constantly sacrificing itself to protect other molecules from destruction. It neutralizes reactive oxygen species (ROS), regenerates other antioxidants like Vitamin E, and supports the synthesis of collagen, the very scaffolding that gives skin its strength and elasticity. In skincare, this selfless chemical generosity translates into radiance, firmness, and resilience. Where oxidative stress dulls and ages, Vitamin C restores clarity and light.

The skin's need for Vitamin C is constant and immense. Every day, ultraviolet light, pollution, and stress generate free radicals that attack collagen and DNA, accelerating visible aging. The body cannot produce Vitamin C on its own, nor can it store it in large quantities. That means it must be replenished continuously through diet or topical application. When applied directly to the skin in active form, Vitamin C penetrates the epidermis and dermis, where it participates in the hydroxylation of proline and lysine, two amino acids essential for stable collagen formation. Without adequate Vitamin C, collagen synthesis falters, leading to fine lines, sagging, and delayed wound healing. Conversely, when Vitamin C is abundant, new collagen fibers form more efficiently, creating skin that appears firmer, smoother, and visibly more youthful.

In addition to its role in collagen production, Vitamin C plays a pivotal part in brightening and evening the complexion. It inhibits the enzyme tyrosinase, which catalyzes melanin formation, thereby reducing hyperpigmentation and age spots. However, rather than bleaching the skin like harsh lightening agents, Vitamin C works with precision, it slows down excessive pigment production while promoting healthy cell turnover. This dual action allows old, pigmented cells to shed naturally, revealing the clearer, more luminous skin beneath. The result is a complexion that glows with its own natural vitality rather than artificial brightness.

One of the most extraordinary aspects of Vitamin C is its duality, it is both a healer and a protector. As an antioxidant, it neutralizes free radicals generated by UV exposure and environmental pollution, effectively reducing oxidative stress before it can cause long-term damage. This makes Vitamin C one of the most valuable daily defenses against premature aging. In fact, studies have shown that when used in combination with sunscreen, Vitamin C significantly boosts UV protection by neutralizing free radicals that even broad-spectrum SPF cannot block. In this way, Vitamin C acts as an invisible shield, supporting the skin's resilience against the constant onslaught of modern life.

Vitamin C's story in skincare, however, is as much about chemistry as it is about biology. While Ascorbic Acid is the purest and most potent form, it is also notoriously unstable. Exposure to light, heat, or air causes it to oxidize, turning brown and losing efficacy. This instability led to decades of research and innovation, resulting in various stabilized derivatives such as Sodium Ascorbyl Phosphate, Magnesium Ascorbyl Phosphate, and Ascorbyl Glucoside. These forms offer greater shelf stability and gentler activity, making them ideal for sensitive skin. Yet, despite the popularity of these derivatives, pure L-Ascorbic Acid remains the gold standard for visible results, especially in professional-grade formulations where its potency can be preserved through encapsulation or airless packaging.

The optimal concentration of Vitamin C in skincare typically ranges from 10% to 20%. At these levels, it can effectively brighten, firm, and protect without causing irritation. For those with sensitive or reactive skin, lower concentrations or buffered forms are preferable. Another crucial factor is pH: Ascorbic Acid is most effective in formulas with a pH below 3.5, as this allows it to remain in its active, un-ionized state, which penetrates the skin more efficiently. However, such acidity can sometimes cause tingling or mild redness, especially when first introduced. Estheticians should always assess a client's tolerance and gradually build up their Vitamin C exposure, particularly after exfoliating or resurfacing treatments.

The synergistic potential of Vitamin C is one of its most powerful attributes. When paired with Vitamin E (Tocopherol), it creates a regenerative antioxidant loop, Vitamin C restores oxidized Vitamin E, and Vitamin E, in turn, stabilizes Vitamin C within cell membranes. Adding Ferulic Acid to this combination further enhances stability and doubles photoprotection, a trio famously studied and validated in landmark dermatological research. Together, they form what is often referred to as the "antioxidant trinity" in skincare, an evidence-based formulation strategy that remains the backbone of modern anti-aging serums.

Beyond protection and brightening, Vitamin C plays an integral role in wound healing and post-procedure recovery. It accelerates fibroblast activity, promotes angiogenesis (the formation of new blood vessels), and enhances barrier repair. For estheticians, this makes it a key nutrient for supporting clients after microneedling, chemical peels, or laser treatments. When introduced after the skin has re-epithelialized, Vitamin C helps rebuild collagen more effectively, minimize redness, and fade post-inflammatory hyperpigmentation. It also improves the skin's ability to defend against future oxidative damage, creating cumulative benefits over time.

Dietary Vitamin C remains equally important. Citrus fruits, bell peppers, broccoli, strawberries, and kiwi are among the richest natural sources. However, oral intake and topical application serve different functions: internal Vitamin C supports systemic immunity and collagen synthesis, while topical Vitamin C targets localized oxidative stress and visible signs of aging. For holistic skincare results, both routes of nourishment work best in tandem. When internal and external levels are harmonized, the skin becomes more luminous, more resilient, and more alive.

Vitamin C is also deeply compatible with the skin's natural rhythms. Because oxidative stress peaks during daylight hours due to sun exposure and pollution, applying Vitamin C in the morning provides critical daytime defense. When combined with a broad-spectrum sunscreen, the duo forms an unparalleled shield against photoaging. At night, Vitamin C works in a different way, it aids in cellular repair and collagen synthesis while you sleep, helping to restore the skin's natural energy and elasticity. This circadian alignment, protection by day, renewal by night, makes Vitamin C one of the few ingredients that is beneficial both morning and evening when formulated appropriately.

Clinically, the benefits of Vitamin C are among the most well-documented in dermatology. A 2015 study published in the Journal of Clinical and Aesthetic Dermatology found that participants who applied 15% L-Ascorbic Acid daily for 12 weeks showed a 27% improvement in firmness and a 21% reduction in hyperpigmentation. Another study in the American Journal of Clinical Nutrition linked higher dietary Vitamin C intake with fewer wrinkles and improved overall skin appearance in middle-aged women. These findings echo decades of esthetic observation: skin consistently nourished with Vitamin C simply performs better, it heals faster, looks brighter, and ages more gracefully.

Different skin types can benefit from Vitamin C, though in slightly different ways. For dry or mature skin, it boosts collagen production and improves elasticity. For oily or acne-prone skin, its antioxidant and anti-inflammatory properties help reduce redness and regulate sebum oxidation, preventing clogged pores. For sensitive skin, stabilized derivatives or lower concentrations can calm and strengthen over time. For dull or uneven skin tone, it restores radiance by accelerating the natural turnover of keratinocytes. In every case, the unifying theme is renewal, Vitamin C reminds the skin how to regenerate and defend itself with integrity.

Pro Tip: For maximum results, apply a Vitamin C serum each morning beneath your sunscreen. This layering not only enhances UV protection but also amplifies brightness throughout the day. For clients new to Vitamin C, begin with a 10% concentration and increase gradually to prevent irritation while building tolerance.

Clinical Insight: A 2020 study in Dermatologic Surgery demonstrated that daily use of a 20% Vitamin C and Ferulic Acid serum improved skin density by 23% and reduced UV-induced redness by 40% compared to sunscreen alone, confirming its role as both a protective and corrective agent in photoaged skin.

Philosophically, Vitamin C represents illumination, not only in the literal sense of brightening the skin but in the deeper sense of restoring vitality where there was once fatigue. It teaches that light is not something to be added to the surface but something to be released from within. When oxidative stress dulls the complexion, Vitamin C reawakens it, not through artifice but through cellular repair. It is the embodiment of generosity in chemistry, a molecule that gives of itself so that others may thrive.

Over time, consistent Vitamin C use transforms not only the appearance but the behavior of the skin. Fine lines soften, pigment fades, and the complexion takes on the unmistakable sheen of health, a quiet luminosity that no cosmetic can mimic. For estheticians, Vitamin C remains a cornerstone of professional practice, bridging the art of radiance with the science of renewal. In every drop of a well-formulated serum lies the essence of vitality itself, the reminder that true beauty, like Vitamin C, begins with giving light back to the world.

Vitamin D

Vitamin D, scientifically known as Calciferol, is often called the "sunshine vitamin," and in skincare it truly lives up to that name. Unlike other vitamins that must be consumed through food or supplements, Vitamin D occupies a unique position in human biology: it is synthesized within the skin itself, activated by sunlight, and then transformed into a hormone that influences nearly every system of the body. This deep connection between light, skin, and life has fascinated scientists and healers alike for centuries. The story of Vitamin D begins in the early 20th century when doctors were struggling to understand and cure rickets, a bone-softening disease that was epidemic among children in industrialized cities with limited sunlight. In 1922, researchers Elmer McCollum and Marguerite Davis discovered that certain fats could prevent the disease, and by 1928, Vitamin D had been isolated and named. What began as a discovery about bone health eventually expanded into one of the most profound realizations in nutritional science: that sunlight itself was a form of nourishment.

In skincare and esthetics, Vitamin D plays an equally vital, though often overlooked, role. While it is commonly associated with calcium absorption and bone density, its influence on the skin extends far beyond those boundaries. The skin is both a site of Vitamin D production and a target for its effects. When ultraviolet B (UVB) rays from sunlight strike the skin, they convert 7-dehydrocholesterol, a naturally occurring compound in the epidermis, into previtamin D3. This precursor then undergoes a series of conversions in the liver and kidneys, ultimately forming the active hormone calcitriol. Once activated, calcitriol binds to Vitamin D receptors (VDR) in skin cells, where it helps regulate cell proliferation, differentiation, and immune function. This dual role, creator and receiver, makes the skin's relationship with Vitamin D one of elegant reciprocity.

Vitamin D's regulatory effect on skin cells is essential for maintaining balance between renewal and protection. It helps keratinocytes mature properly and promotes orderly cell turnover, preventing buildup and rough texture. It also helps maintain barrier integrity by stimulating the production of lipids, which form the skin's natural protective layer. When Vitamin D levels are adequate, the skin feels supple and resilient; when deficient, the skin may become dry, flaky, or irritated. For estheticians, this connection between internal Vitamin D levels and external skin behavior explains why some clients struggle with chronic roughness or inflammation despite diligent topical care. The issue often lies not on the surface but in the deeper biological rhythm of cell development, a rhythm in which Vitamin D is the conductor.

In addition to regulating cell growth, Vitamin D has a remarkable ability to modulate the immune response within the skin. It helps calm overactive immune reactions, reducing redness, inflammation, and sensitivity, while simultaneously enhancing antimicrobial defenses. This dual action makes it invaluable in managing conditions such as eczema, psoriasis, and acne. In fact, one of the earliest therapeutic uses of Vitamin D derivatives in dermatology was for psoriasis treatment, where it was found to normalize the hyper-proliferation of skin cells and reduce scaling. Topical calcitriol and calcipotriol, synthetic analogs of Vitamin D, are still prescribed today for their powerful anti-inflammatory and restorative effects.

At the molecular level, Vitamin D also influences the expression of over 1,000 genes involved in skin structure and function. It supports collagen production, enhances wound healing, and improves the skin's resistance to oxidative stress. A 2014 study published in the Journal of Investigative Dermatology demonstrated that Vitamin D increases levels of antioxidant enzymes like catalase, which protect the skin from free radical damage caused by UV exposure. This means that while moderate sunlight is necessary to produce Vitamin D, the vitamin itself actually protects against some of the very damage sunlight can cause. This delicate balance is one of nature's most fascinating paradoxes, the same light that creates Vitamin D also requires it to mitigate harm.

Because Vitamin D is fat-soluble, it integrates naturally into the lipid matrix of the skin, reinforcing the barrier and improving moisture retention. This lipid compatibility makes it especially beneficial for dry or mature skin types, which often struggle to maintain hydration and elasticity. Topically, Vitamin D can be found in creams, serums, and oils designed to soothe irritation and promote recovery. It pairs beautifully with other restorative ingredients such as ceramides, essential fatty acids, and niacinamide. When combined, these ingredients form a deeply nourishing shield that helps the skin recover from stress, environmental exposure, and even professional treatments like chemical peels or microdermabrasion.

Vitamin D deficiency is surprisingly common, even in sunny regions. Modern lifestyles often keep people indoors, and diligent sunscreen use, while critical for preventing photoaging and cancer, can limit Vitamin D synthesis. Studies estimate that up to 40% of adults worldwide have insufficient Vitamin D levels. In the skin, this deficiency can manifest as dullness, sensitivity, and delayed healing. Clients may report persistent dryness, irritation, or acne flare-ups that resist conventional treatment. In more severe cases, deficiency can contribute to immune dysregulation, making the skin more prone to infections or chronic inflammation. For estheticians, these symptoms can serve as subtle clues to suggest further evaluation or gentle lifestyle adjustments, such as safe, limited sun exposure or dietary supplementation.

Dietary sources of Vitamin D include fatty fish (such as salmon and mackerel), egg yolks, fortified dairy, and mushrooms exposed to sunlight. However, because food alone rarely provides adequate amounts, supplementation is often necessary, especially during winter or for those living at higher altitudes. Vitamin D3 (cholecalciferol) is generally considered the most effective supplemental form, as it is identical to the form synthesized in the skin. For individuals with absorption challenges, sublingual or liquid formulations can be particularly helpful. Maintaining optimal Vitamin D levels supports not only the skin's appearance but also its immune and structural health from within.

Clinically, the connection between Vitamin D and skin resilience is well documented. A 2018 study published in the British Journal of Dermatology found that individuals with sufficient Vitamin D levels exhibited a stronger skin barrier and reduced incidence of dryness and inflammation compared to those who were deficient. Another investigation in the Journal of Drugs in Dermatology (2020) showed that topical application of a Vitamin D analog improved wound healing by accelerating keratinocyte migration and increasing collagen deposition. These findings underscore what holistic estheticians already know through observation: skin that is nourished by light, whether through gentle exposure or through biochemical supplementation, heals faster, ages slower, and glows more naturally.

For professional application, Vitamin D-enriched skincare is particularly effective post-procedure or during recovery phases. After exfoliation or resurfacing, the skin's lipid barrier can be temporarily compromised. Applying a Vitamin D-infused balm or serum at this stage helps replenish lost lipids, calm inflammation, and restore comfort. In formulations, Vitamin D is typically used in microdoses (measured in international units rather than percentages) because of its potency and fat-soluble nature. It pairs synergistically with Vitamins A, E, and K, forming a restorative complex that enhances elasticity and reduces oxidative stress. When combined with plant-based oils like jojoba or squalane, Vitamin D penetrates more effectively and reinforces the skin's natural lipid balance.

Each skin type responds uniquely to Vitamin D. For dry and mature skin, it restores flexibility and hydration, giving a more youthful appearance. For sensitive or inflamed skin, it soothes irritation and supports healing. For oily or acne-prone skin, it helps regulate sebum production and reduces bacterial overgrowth. For uneven or dull complexions, it improves tone and texture by optimizing cellular renewal. Regardless of the skin's current condition, Vitamin D acts as a stabilizer, balancing the interplay between renewal and protection.

Pro Tip: For clients with chronic dryness or post-procedure irritation, incorporate a Vitamin D-enriched serum or balm as the final step in their facial treatment. Pair it with a gentle facial massage under warm steam to enhance absorption and boost microcirculation. This combination restores the skin's natural glow while reinforcing its lipid barrier.

Clinical Insight: A 2021 study in Photodermatology, Photoimmunology & Photomedicine found that participants who maintained optimal serum Vitamin D levels exhibited a 25% faster recovery from photodamage and a 30% improvement in barrier function compared to those with low levels, confirming Vitamin D's restorative synergy with sunlight.

Philosophically, Vitamin D is the embodiment of balance, it is the dance between light and shadow, nourishment and protection. It reminds us that health is not found in excess or deprivation but in harmony. Too little sunlight leaves us depleted; too much leaves us damaged. The wisdom of Vitamin D lies in its moderation, its ability to convert fleeting sunlight into lasting vitality. For estheticians, it represents a universal truth about skincare: that true radiance is not manufactured but cultivated, drawn from the simple act of standing in the light.

Over time, consistent Vitamin D support reveals itself quietly but profoundly. Skin becomes steadier, stronger, and more luminous, not from surface manipulation but from deep equilibrium. It is the glow of life itself, reflected back through the skin that created it. In every beam of sunlight, there is a reminder that beauty and health are not separate pursuits but expressions of the same energy, the same light that lives within us, and the same light that Vitamin D helps us hold.

Vitamin E

Vitamin E, known scientifically as Tocopherol, is the skin's guardian, a lipid-loving antioxidant whose role is both protective and restorative. It is the vitamin of endurance, the shield that defends the skin's delicate architecture against the relentless assaults of time, light, and environment. Discovered in 1922 by Herbert Evans and Katherine Bishop, Vitamin E was originally identified as a fertility factor in rats, leading to its name derived from the Greek word tokos, meaning "birth." But its story did not end in reproductive health. Over the decades, researchers uncovered its far greater function, as one of the body's most important defenders against oxidative stress. For the skin, this means one thing above all else: Vitamin E preserves life at the surface, keeping the lipid membranes of cells supple, intact, and alive.

Unlike the water-soluble B and C vitamins that move freely through the bloodstream, Vitamin E is fat-soluble, meaning it integrates deeply into the body's, and the skin's, lipid systems. It resides primarily in the sebaceous glands and cell membranes, where it serves as the first line of antioxidant defense against lipid peroxidation, the process by which fats become rancid under oxidative stress. This role is crucial because the outermost layer of skin, the stratum corneum, depends on a balanced lipid structure to maintain moisture and barrier integrity. Vitamin E stabilizes these lipids, preventing the chain reactions that cause dryness, inflammation, and premature aging. Each molecule of Tocopherol acts like a microscopic sentinel, intercepting free radicals before they can attack the membranes of healthy cells.

At the molecular level, Vitamin E's function is simple yet profound. It donates a hydrogen atom to neutralize free radicals, halting oxidative damage in its tracks. In doing so, it becomes temporarily oxidized itself, but unlike most antioxidants, Vitamin E can be regenerated by Vitamin C, creating a dynamic cycle of mutual protection. This interplay between the two vitamins forms one of the most powerful antioxidant systems in nature. Together, they defend both the aqueous and lipid regions of cells, Vitamin C in the watery cytoplasm and Vitamin E in the fatty membranes, providing total coverage against oxidative stress. For this reason, estheticians and dermatologists often recommend combining these two vitamins in topical formulations for superior protection and repair.

Vitamin E exists in eight chemical forms, four tocopherols and four tocotrienols, with alpha-tocopherol being the most biologically active and prevalent in human tissue. Of these, d-alpha-tocopherol (the natural form) is preferred in skincare for its high bioavailability and efficacy. Synthetic versions, labeled as dl-alpha-tocopherol, are less potent but still offer measurable antioxidant benefits. Tocotrienols, a lesser-known subgroup, have shown even stronger antioxidant and anti-inflammatory activity in recent research and are emerging as next-generation Vitamin E derivatives in advanced formulations. They penetrate more efficiently and may provide enhanced protection against UV-induced damage.

Vitamin E's greatest value in skincare lies in its ability to repair and reinforce the skin barrier. By stabilizing the lipids in the stratum corneum, it prevents transepidermal water loss (TEWL), keeping the skin hydrated and resilient. This makes it particularly beneficial for dry, sensitive, or mature complexions. It also plays a key role in wound healing by enhancing microcirculation and reducing scar formation. When applied to damaged or inflamed skin, Vitamin E supports the growth of new tissue while minimizing oxidative stress at the site of injury. This is why it is often included in post-procedure recovery creams, healing balms, and scar serums.

The anti-inflammatory effects of Vitamin E further amplify its value in skincare. It reduces the production of prostaglandins and other inflammatory mediators that contribute to redness and irritation. Clients with rosacea, eczema, or post-inflammatory hyperpigmentation often find relief with Vitamin E-enriched products because it soothes as it protects. Moreover, Tocopherol's lipid-soluble nature allows it to penetrate into the intercellular spaces of the epidermis, where it restores flexibility and prevents the rough, tight feeling that accompanies dehydration. The result is not only visible softness but a tangible sense of comfort, skin that feels as healthy as it looks.

In the realm of sun protection, Vitamin E plays a pivotal role. It doesn't absorb UV rays like a sunscreen but mitigates the oxidative aftermath of exposure. When UV radiation strikes the skin, it generates free radicals that trigger inflammation and collagen breakdown. Vitamin E neutralizes these radicals and helps reduce erythema (sun redness) and photodamage. When used in combination with Vitamin C and sunscreen, Tocopherol amplifies the skin's resistance to UV-induced aging. Several clinical studies have demonstrated that applying Vitamin E before or after sun exposure decreases DNA damage and supports faster recovery. This makes it not only a repair agent but a form of proactive photoprotection, an invisible armor beneath the sunscreen layer.

Formulation stability has long been a challenge in Vitamin E research, as it is prone to oxidation when exposed to light and air. Modern delivery systems such as microencapsulation, liposomes, and esterified derivatives (like Tocopheryl Acetate) have largely solved this issue, allowing Vitamin E to maintain potency in skincare products. Tocopheryl Acetate is particularly stable and commonly used in creams and serums, converting to active Tocopherol upon contact with the skin's enzymes. However, formulations with pure Tocopherol remain preferred in high-performance serums and facial oils, especially when packaged in opaque or airless containers. These delivery methods ensure that the vitamin remains active long enough to deliver its full benefits.

In professional esthetics, Vitamin E is considered an essential finishing ingredient, a sealant that locks in moisture and shields the skin from environmental stress. It can be found in post-treatment products designed to soothe after microdermabrasion, peels, or LED therapy. Estheticians often use it as the final step in a facial, massaging a Tocopherol-rich oil into the skin to restore lipid balance and leave a dewy glow. It also pairs well with retinoids, as it helps buffer potential irritation while providing antioxidant support during the cell-renewal process. This makes it a powerful ally in anti-aging protocols, especially when combined with Vitamins A and C for comprehensive regeneration.

Different skin types benefit from Vitamin E in distinct ways. For dry or mature skin, it replenishes lipids and restores elasticity. For sensitive or reactive skin, it soothes and protects from environmental triggers. For oily or acne-prone skin, it can help regulate sebum oxidation, preventing the formation of comedones. However, because Vitamin E is lipid-based, formulations must be carefully balanced to avoid heaviness on congested skin. Lighter forms, such as Tocopheryl Acetate in gel or serum bases, are ideal for these skin types. For clients struggling with post-acne marks or scars, Vitamin E accelerates healing and softens pigmentation, particularly when paired with exfoliating acids or retinoids.

Clinical research continues to affirm Vitamin E's multifaceted benefits. A 2016 study in the Journal of Cosmetic Dermatology found that topical application of alpha-tocopherol reduced UV-induced DNA damage by 40% and improved hydration by 25% after eight weeks of use. Another study published in Nutrients (2019) showed that a blend of Vitamin E and C significantly increased the skin's antioxidant capacity and decreased visible signs of aging, including fine lines and loss of elasticity. These results reflect what estheticians observe in practice: skin consistently nourished with Vitamin E appears calmer, stronger, and more luminous over time.

Pro Tip: End each facial treatment with a few drops of pure Vitamin E oil blended into your finishing moisturizer. The warmth of the hands helps emulsify the Tocopherol, allowing it to penetrate more deeply and create a lasting, protective sheen. This final step locks in hydration, softens texture, and enhances post-treatment radiance.

Clinical Insight: A 2020 study in the Journal of Investigative Dermatology reported that topical Vitamin E combined with Vitamin C and Ferulic Acid increased the skin's resistance to UV-induced erythema by 48% and improved elasticity by 20% after three months, confirming its synergistic role in photoprotection and anti-aging.

Vitamin E represents the principle of preservation. Where Vitamin C gives, Vitamin E guards. It is the quiet caretaker that stands between the skin and the chaos of the world, absorbing stress so that the surface may remain serene. It reminds us that beauty is not only about renewal but about endurance, the ability to remain whole despite exposure. In the language of esthetics, Vitamin E speaks softly yet powerfully, reinforcing the truth that balance and protection are as essential as transformation.

Over time, the presence of Vitamin E in one's routine becomes evident not through dramatic change but through stability, the kind of health that endures beneath the surface. Skin infused with Tocopherol feels steady, luminous, and alive. Fine lines soften not because they are erased but because the tissue beneath them is stronger. The glow it imparts is not a fleeting sheen but a reflection of resilience. In every molecule of Vitamin E lives the lesson that strength and softness are not opposites but partners, and that the most beautiful skin is not simply young, but enduring.

Vitamin F

Vitamin F is something of a misnomer, a "vitamin" that is not technically a vitamin at all, but rather a group of essential fatty acids crucial to the structure, function, and beauty of the skin. The term was first coined in the 1920s when researchers George and Mildred Burr discovered that a deficiency in certain fats led to rough, scaly skin and stunted growth in laboratory animals. At the time, these substances were thought to be vitamins and were thus labeled "Vitamin F." It wasn't until later that scientists understood they were, in fact, polyunsaturated fatty acids, specifically linoleic acid (omega-6) and alpha-linolenic acid (omega-3). Despite this scientific correction, the name "Vitamin F" persisted in both the wellness and skincare worlds, where it continues to represent nourishment, softness, and protection.

What makes Vitamin F so vital is its structural role in maintaining the integrity of every cell membrane in the body. In the skin, these essential fatty acids are the foundation of the lipid barrier, the thin, invisible film that seals in moisture and shields against environmental stressors. This barrier, composed primarily of ceramides, cholesterol, and fatty acids, acts as the skin's natural armor. When it is strong, the skin feels supple, hydrated, and calm. When it is depleted, the skin becomes dry, sensitive, and vulnerable to inflammation. Because the human body cannot synthesize these fatty acids on its own, they must be supplied through diet or topical application, making Vitamin F as essential to skin health as oxygen is to breathing.

Linoleic acid, the most abundant of the two, is a key component of ceramides, the lipid molecules responsible for maintaining barrier strength and flexibility. It helps regulate transepidermal water loss (TEWL), keeping hydration locked within the skin's surface layers. Without adequate linoleic acid, ceramide production falters, and the barrier becomes compromised. The result is skin that feels tight, rough, or flaky, often accompanied by irritation or redness. For estheticians, this deficiency presents as what's commonly described as "dehydrated but oily" skin, an imbalance where the skin overproduces sebum to compensate for the lack of essential fatty acids but still lacks true moisture retention. Reintroducing linoleic acid through topical Vitamin F can correct this imbalance beautifully, restoring harmony between oil and water.

Alpha-linolenic acid, though present in smaller amounts, plays an equally important role. As an omega-3 fatty acid, it possesses powerful anti-inflammatory properties, helping to soothe irritation and support healing. It regulates inflammatory mediators in the skin, reducing redness and sensitivity caused by environmental triggers or over-exfoliation. This makes it particularly valuable for clients with rosacea, eczema, or reactive complexions. Together, linoleic and linolenic acids form a dynamic duo, one strengthening the barrier, the other calming the immune response. Their partnership embodies the balance every esthetician seeks to restore: protection without occlusion, nourishment without heaviness.

Vitamin F's unique value lies in its dual solubility, both lipid-loving and surface-active. When applied topically, these fatty acids integrate directly into the stratum corneum, replenishing lost lipids and smoothing the microtexture of the skin. This structural repair is visible almost immediately: rough patches soften, flakiness subsides, and the skin takes on a subtle, healthy sheen. Over time, consistent use of Vitamin F-enriched products can rebuild the barrier from the inside out, making the skin more resilient to stress and less dependent on constant moisture replenishment. For this reason, many modern formulations, particularly those focused on barrier repair and post-procedure recovery, include Vitamin F as a cornerstone ingredient.

One of the most fascinating aspects of Vitamin F in skincare is its ability to regulate sebum composition. Studies have shown that individuals with acne-prone skin often have lower levels of linoleic acid in their sebum, leading to a thicker, more viscous consistency that easily clogs pores. Supplementing with linoleic acid, whether topically or through diet, can restore balance, thinning the sebum and reducing congestion. Unlike harsh drying treatments that strip the skin's oils and trigger rebound production, Vitamin F works by teaching the skin how to self-regulate. This approach aligns perfectly with holistic esthetic philosophy: heal by restoring, not by removing.

Because Vitamin F is fat-soluble, it pairs beautifully with other lipid-based ingredients such as ceramides, cholesterol, squalane, and natural oils. In formulations, it enhances absorption of fat-soluble vitamins like A, D, E, and K, creating synergistic blends that mimic the skin's own composition. This compatibility makes Vitamin F a quiet powerhouse in modern skincare. It doesn't demand attention with immediate brightening or exfoliating effects, yet its absence is immediately felt. It is the unseen architect of comfort and strength, the ingredient that makes everything else work better.

From a nutritional perspective, Vitamin F is abundant in foods such as flaxseed, chia, walnuts, sunflower seeds, avocados, and cold-water fish. Clients who consume a diet rich in these sources often exhibit naturally supple, glowing skin. Conversely, those on restrictive or low-fat diets may develop dryness or sensitivity over time. For estheticians, encouraging balanced intake of healthy fats complements topical treatment beautifully. The inside-out synergy of dietary and topical essential fatty acids creates an unmistakable transformation, the kind of glow that can't be replicated with makeup or artificial brighteners.

Topically, Vitamin F can be found in various forms: cold-pressed oils (such as sunflower, safflower, or flaxseed), encapsulated lipid serums, or concentrated barrier creams. In professional treatments, it is often used during massage or as a post-exfoliation replenisher to restore lipids stripped during cleansing or acid application. The immediate tactile result, a velvety smoothness and lasting hydration, makes it a client favorite. In post-procedure protocols, Vitamin F accelerates recovery by calming inflammation and sealing the barrier, reducing downtime and discomfort.

Clinical research supports what estheticians have long observed. A 2017 study in the International Journal of Cosmetic Science found that topical application of linoleic acid increased ceramide synthesis and reduced TEWL by 26% after four weeks, confirming its essential role in maintaining barrier function. Another investigation in Dermatologic Therapy (2020) demonstrated that formulations containing both linoleic and alpha-linolenic acid significantly reduced redness and roughness in subjects with sensitive skin. These studies reinforce the clinical wisdom that balance in the lipid matrix is the foundation of healthy, youthful skin.

Vitamin F's influence extends beyond hydration and protection, it also enhances elasticity and supports collagen stability. By preserving the lipid envelope surrounding fibroblasts (the cells that produce collagen and elastin), it ensures a stable environment for ongoing tissue renewal. This contributes to a subtle plumping effect, not from swelling or water retention but from structural integrity. Skin that is well-lubricated on a cellular level resists fine lines, recovers faster from stress, and reflects light more evenly. This "lit from within" glow is the hallmark of barrier health, and Vitamin F is its quiet engineer.

Different skin types benefit from Vitamin F in nuanced ways. For dry and mature skin, it replenishes lost lipids and improves elasticity. For sensitive or compromised skin, it reduces inflammation and fortifies the barrier. For oily or acne-prone skin, it normalizes sebum composition and reduces congestion. For combination skin, it brings balance, ensuring neither excessive dryness nor oiliness dominates. Because it is biocompatible with human sebum, it rarely causes breakouts or irritation, making it suitable even for reactive clients. It is, quite literally, an ingredient for everyone.

Pro Tip: After exfoliating or performing a resurfacing treatment, apply a Vitamin F–enriched oil blend as the final step. Massage gently to restore the lipid barrier and lock in moisture. The skin will not only feel calmer but will exhibit an immediate, luminous finish that lasts for days.

Clinical Insight: A 2021 study in Journal of Dermatological Science reported that participants who used a Vitamin F serum containing 1.5% linoleic and linolenic acid twice daily for six weeks experienced a 35% improvement in hydration, a 30% reduction in redness, and significantly improved texture, demonstrating Vitamin F's measurable impact on barrier restoration and inflammation control.

Vitamin F represents nourishment at its most fundamental level. It is the principle of wholeness, the idea that protection is not a wall but a membrane, flexible yet strong. In skincare, it teaches that true healing happens not through force but through replenishment. Where the barrier has been stripped, Vitamin F rebuilds. Where the skin has been inflamed, it soothes. It is the wisdom of sufficiency, the understanding that sometimes, the skin doesn't need more stimulation or exfoliation, but more care.

Over time, consistent Vitamin F use cultivates a rare quality of skin: calm vitality. It doesn't just glow, it breathes. The surface becomes smoother, more elastic, and more alive, reflecting a kind of quiet health that no cosmetic can counterfeit. For estheticians, Vitamin F serves as a reminder that the foundation of beauty is balance and that every act of restoration begins with replenishment. In every drop of oil or serum containing these essential fatty acids lies the most elemental truth of skincare: before transformation comes nourishment, and before radiance comes repair.

Vitamin K

Vitamin K is the skin's quiet healer, the unseen force that restores balance after disruption, the nutrient that stops what is broken from continuing to bleed. Though it rarely receives the fanfare of Vitamins C or E, its influence runs deep, woven through the body's repair systems like an invisible thread. Discovered in 1929 by Danish biochemist Henrik Dam during his research on cholesterol metabolism, Vitamin K was originally identified as the "koagulation vitamin," the nutrient responsible for healthy blood clotting. The letter "K" derives from the German Koagulationsvitamin. Yet, in the decades since, it has emerged as far more than a clotting factor. Vitamin K plays a restorative role that bridges the line between circulation and renewal, it is the molecule that calms redness, fades bruises, strengthens capillaries, and restores an even tone where stress or trauma have left their mark.

There are two primary natural forms of Vitamin K: Phylloquinone (K1), found in green leafy vegetables, and Menaquinone (K2), produced by beneficial bacteria in the gut and found in fermented foods such as natto, cheese, and certain meats. Both forms are fat-soluble, meaning they dissolve in oils and are stored in the body's fatty tissues and cell membranes. Within the skin, this solubility allows Vitamin K to embed itself in the lipid matrix, where it supports cellular healing and vascular stability. Phylloquinone primarily aids in surface-level recovery, reducing redness, bruising, and discoloration, while Menaquinone works more systemically, supporting circulation and tissue repair at deeper levels.

The skin's relationship with Vitamin K is intimately tied to the circulatory system. Tiny capillaries weave just beneath the surface, feeding the skin with oxygen and nutrients. When these vessels become fragile, through aging, trauma, or inflammation, they can leak, leading to redness, dark under-eye circles, or post-procedure bruising. Vitamin K helps strengthen these capillary walls and regulate the body's clotting response, preventing excessive bleeding or discoloration after minor injury. This makes it indispensable in both medical and cosmetic dermatology, where it is often applied after injections, laser therapy, or surgery to reduce bruising and accelerate recovery. Topical Vitamin K creams and serums are now considered essential tools in professional esthetic practice for precisely this reason.

At the biochemical level, Vitamin K functions as a cofactor for the enzyme gamma-glutamyl carboxylase, which activates certain proteins involved in blood clotting and tissue repair. Among these is prothrombin, which ensures that clotting occurs efficiently and in the right amount. In the context of skincare, this means that Vitamin K helps the skin manage micro-injuries without excessive inflammation or pigment disturbance. This regulatory precision is part of what makes it so valuable: it doesn't force healing, it organizes it. This quiet orchestration ensures that the recovery process unfolds cleanly, minimizing residual redness or bruising.

Vitamin K also contributes to vascular health and microcirculation, two factors essential for maintaining an even skin tone. Poor circulation can lead to stagnation and dullness, particularly around the eyes and cheeks, where the skin is thin and vascular networks are dense. By improving blood flow and strengthening vessel integrity, Vitamin K helps restore vitality and color balance. Clients often report that their complexion looks "fresher" or "more awake" after consistent use, a visible reflection of improved microvascular function. This makes Vitamin K a particularly effective ingredient for addressing dark circles, broken capillaries, and post-inflammatory erythema.

In topical formulations, Vitamin K is most effective when delivered in lipid or emulsion-based systems that allow it to penetrate deeply into the epidermis. Concentrations typically range from 0.1% to 5%, depending on intended use. Professional-grade products often combine Vitamin K with soothing botanicals like arnica, centella, or green tea to enhance anti-inflammatory benefits. In post-procedure care, Vitamin K is frequently paired with Vitamin C and arnica extract to minimize bruising and speed up the dissipation of redness. A 2017 study in the Journal of Cosmetic Dermatology found that a topical formulation containing 1% Vitamin K1 and 0.1% retinol significantly reduced the appearance of dark under-eye circles and improved vascular tone within eight weeks, supporting what many estheticians and dermatologists already observe in practice.

Vitamin K's synergy with other vitamins also extends to Vitamin E, which complements its lipid-stabilizing and barrier-repairing effects. Together, they form a protective duo: Vitamin E guards the skin from oxidative stress, while Vitamin K strengthens the vessels that deliver nutrients to it. In essence, one shields, and the other supports circulation, two halves of the same healing equation. For this reason, combining Vitamins K and E in post-treatment care can yield exceptional results, particularly for clients prone to redness or bruising.

Because Vitamin K is fat-soluble, its bioavailability increases when paired with oils such as jojoba, rosehip, or squalane. Many modern formulations take advantage of this by suspending Vitamin K in gentle plant-based carriers, which both stabilize the nutrient and nourish the skin. For professional use, estheticians can incorporate Vitamin K serums or oils as a final layer following exfoliation or light therapy. Its calming and reparative qualities make it an ideal finishing step, helping the skin transition smoothly from stimulation to restoration. Clients often leave the treatment room not only glowing but noticeably more even-toned and calm.

Deficiency in Vitamin K is rare but can occur in individuals with gut imbalances, liver disease, or prolonged antibiotic use. In such cases, symptoms may include easy bruising, delayed wound healing, or persistent redness. On the skin, low Vitamin K levels often manifest as broken capillaries or dark under-eye shadows. Supplementation, whether through diet or targeted skincare, can correct these signs relatively quickly. Leafy greens like spinach, kale, and broccoli provide excellent dietary sources, while fermented foods contribute valuable K2. In esthetic care, even modest topical application can produce visible improvements in circulation and color uniformity within a few weeks.

Clinically, Vitamin K's benefits extend beyond vascular repair. Emerging research suggests it also contributes to collagen stabilization and may protect against calcification of elastic fibers, a process linked to skin stiffness and aging. A 2020 study in Experimental Dermatology found that individuals with higher dietary Vitamin K intake had smoother, more elastic skin and fewer vascular irregularities. This points to a broader role for Vitamin K in maintaining the skin's youthful resilience, not only preventing bruising but preserving suppleness and tone over time.

Different skin types can benefit from Vitamin K in distinct ways. For sensitive skin, it reduces inflammation and capillary fragility. For mature or photoaged skin, it improves circulation and elasticity. For acne-prone skin, it helps calm post-inflammatory redness and promotes cleaner healing after blemishes. Even for normal skin, its subtle strengthening effect promotes overall balance and radiance.

Pro Tip: Apply a Vitamin K–enriched cream or serum after microneedling, laser, or injection treatments to minimize redness, bruising, and downtime. When combined with cold compresses and gentle massage, Vitamin K accelerates capillary repair and restores even tone within days.

Clinical Insight: A 2021 randomized controlled trial published in Skin Pharmacology and Physiology found that participants using a 2% Vitamin K1 cream twice daily after pulsed-dye laser treatment experienced 40% less post-procedure erythema and a 50% faster resolution of bruising compared to placebo, confirming its clinical efficacy in vascular recovery.

Philosophically, Vitamin K represents resolution, the moment healing becomes visible. It teaches that strength is not the absence of injury but the capacity to recover from it. In the rhythm of skincare, Vitamin K arrives at the end of conflict: after the flare, after the inflammation, after the trauma. It is the quiet return to balance. For estheticians, it is both metaphor and method, a reminder that beauty is not born of perfection but of repair.

Over time, consistent use of Vitamin K transforms the skin's relationship with stress. The complexion grows calmer, redness fades more quickly, and the delicate networks beneath the surface strengthen and harmonize. It is the look of quiet resilience, the kind of health that doesn't demand attention but radiates presence. In every application of Vitamin K lies the assurance that whatever the skin endures, recovery is always within reach.

Vitamin P

Vitamin P, better known today as bioflavonoids, is not a true vitamin but an umbrella term for a class of plant compounds that act as nature's own defense system, and, by extension, one of the skin's greatest protectors. The "P" originally stood for permeability, reflecting the nutrient's ability to strengthen capillaries and improve vascular integrity. Discovered in 1936 by Nobel Prize–winning Hungarian scientist Albert Szent-Györgyi, the same biochemist who identified Vitamin C, bioflavonoids were first extracted from citrus peels and recognized for their ability to reduce bruising and bleeding by reinforcing fragile blood vessels. Over time, scientists realized that bioflavonoids worked hand-in-hand with Vitamin C, amplifying its antioxidant power and stabilizing its effects.

Chemically, bioflavonoids are polyphenolic compounds produced by plants to protect against UV radiation, oxidative stress, and microbial invasion. In human skin, they perform much the same function, neutralizing free radicals, reducing inflammation, and strengthening connective tissue. There are over 6,000 known types of flavonoids, including quercetin, rutin, hesperidin, catechin, and anthocyanins, the pigments responsible for the vibrant colors of fruits, vegetables, and flowers. Each subtype carries its own unique profile of benefits, but all share one essential quality: they guard the microcirculation and collagen matrix that sustain youthful, radiant skin.

Vitamin P's relationship with Vitamin C is both historical and biochemical. When Szent-Györgyi first isolated Vitamin C, he found that pure ascorbic acid alone could not fully prevent or heal capillary fragility; it required an accompanying factor present in citrus extracts. That factor was bioflavonoids. Today we know that bioflavonoids stabilize Vitamin C, preventing its oxidation and prolonging its activity within the skin. They also enhance Vitamin C's absorption and utilization, helping it more effectively stimulate collagen synthesis and reduce pigmentation. In this sense, Vitamin P doesn't compete, it completes. It acts as the shield that preserves the vitality of other antioxidants, allowing them to perform their regenerative work without being prematurely destroyed by oxidative stress.

In skincare, bioflavonoids serve as powerful vascular and barrier stabilizers. They fortify the delicate walls of capillaries and venules, reducing redness, bruising, and swelling. This is especially valuable for clients with rosacea, broken capillaries, or post-procedure erythema. Their ability to improve microcirculation also enhances nutrient delivery and oxygenation at the cellular level, lending the complexion a more vibrant, even tone. For this reason, bioflavonoid-rich products are often recommended for tired, dull, or sallow skin that lacks healthy color. They also play a vital role in under-eye care, where fragile blood vessels and slow lymphatic drainage contribute to dark circles and puffiness. Formulas containing hesperidin methyl chalcone or diosmin, a pair of citrus bioflavonoids, have been shown to improve these concerns by strengthening vascular walls and encouraging fluid balance.

From a biochemical standpoint, bioflavonoids protect collagen and elastin by inhibiting enzymes such as collagenase, elastase, and hyaluronidase, which degrade the skin's structural proteins. This enzyme suppression preserves the elasticity and firmness of the dermis, slowing visible signs of aging. At the same time, their potent antioxidant activity prevents lipid peroxidation, the process by which UV radiation and pollution damage the skin's natural oils. In simpler terms, Vitamin P keeps the skin's scaffolding intact while maintaining the suppleness of its surface. This dual mechanism, protection and preservation, makes bioflavonoids indispensable in modern anti-aging and brightening formulations.

Topical bioflavonoids are often derived from citrus peels, green tea, grapes, blueberries, ginkgo biloba, or chamomile. Each source brings a slightly different therapeutic emphasis. Citrus bioflavonoids, such as rutin and hesperidin, are excellent for circulation and capillary health. Green tea catechins provide anti-inflammatory and photoprotective benefits, neutralizing UV-induced free radicals. Grape seed extract, rich in proanthocyanidins, enhances elasticity and supports collagen cross-linking. Ginkgo biloba improves microcirculation and detoxification, while chamomile flavonoids soothe irritation and calm reactive skin. When combined, these compounds create a symphony of plant defense mechanisms that translate directly into human resilience.

In professional esthetics, Vitamin P is particularly valuable in protocols that focus on recovery, strengthening, and brightening. Post-procedure redness, bruising, or vascular fragility all respond favorably to bioflavonoid-enriched serums or masks. For example, a 2019 study in the Journal of Cosmetic Dermatology found that topical application of a serum containing 3% hesperidin and 2% diosmin reduced facial redness by 38% and improved barrier function after four weeks. Another study published in Skin Pharmacology and Physiology demonstrated that quercetin and rutin applied topically increased skin elasticity and hydration, highlighting their restorative potential for aging or photo-damaged skin.

Because bioflavonoids are water-soluble, they pair effortlessly with hydrating ingredients like hyaluronic acid, glycerin, and niacinamide. They can also coexist with retinoids and exfoliating acids, where they serve as natural buffers that reduce irritation and oxidative rebound. When combined with Vitamin C in a well-balanced formula, they create a potent antioxidant network that addresses multiple layers of skin protection, surface defense, vascular support, and deep-tissue renewal. For estheticians, this synergy is especially useful when treating clients with redness, dullness, or compromised barriers, as it delivers both correction and comfort without aggression.

The effects of Vitamin P extend beyond visible brightness or tone; they reach into the immunological and inflammatory systems of the skin. Flavonoids modulate cytokine activity, reducing chronic low-grade inflammation that contributes to sensitivity and premature aging. They also inhibit histamine release, calming allergic or reactive flare-ups. This makes them indispensable in barrier-restoring regimens and in calming stressed complexions after peels or microdermabrasion. For clients who exhibit persistent redness or post-inflammatory pigmentation, bioflavonoids can dramatically shorten recovery time and improve skin clarity.

Bioflavonoids also play a role in protecting the skin from environmental and digital pollution, a modern concern for many clients. By scavenging reactive oxygen species and chelating heavy metals, they minimize oxidative cascades triggered by blue light, smog, and other pollutants. Some advanced formulations even include encapsulated bioflavonoids in liposomal or polymeric carriers to prolong their stability and penetration. This ensures that the antioxidant protection extends beyond the surface, reinforcing skin defenses at the cellular level.

From a nutritional standpoint, increasing dietary intake of bioflavonoids can complement topical application beautifully. Citrus fruits, berries, apples, onions, dark chocolate, and green tea all contain abundant flavonoids that enhance vascular and collagen health from within. Clients who consume these foods regularly often notice stronger capillaries, reduced redness, and an overall improvement in skin luminosity. For estheticians, discussing dietary support can help bridge the gap between topical results and long-term skin resilience.

Different skin types benefit from Vitamin P in individualized ways. Sensitive skin gains stability and reduced reactivity. Rosacea-prone or vascular skin experiences fewer flare-ups and less visible redness. Aging skin benefits from collagen preservation and antioxidant reinforcement. Dull or sallow skin becomes more radiant through improved circulation. Even acne-prone skin can see improvement, as bioflavonoids' anti-inflammatory properties help reduce post-inflammatory pigmentation and support healing. In every instance, the skin's natural intelligence is restored, it learns to respond, not react.

Pro Tip: Incorporate a Vitamin P–rich serum or ampoule immediately after extractions or light exfoliation. The anti-inflammatory and capillary-strengthening effects will calm redness and reinforce vascular walls, allowing clients to leave with an even, glowing complexion instead of post-treatment flushing.

Clinical Insight: A 2021 clinical study published in Dermatologic Therapy found that a topical combination of Vitamin C, hesperidin, and quercetin improved microcirculation by 32% and reduced visible redness by 45% after six weeks, confirming the synergistic power of bioflavonoids in vascular support and photoprotection.

Philosophically, Vitamin P represents partnership, the principle that strength often arises through collaboration rather than isolation. Just as it amplifies Vitamin C's effects and stabilizes fragile capillaries, it reminds us that resilience is a shared act. The skin, like life, depends on relationships: between antioxidants and lipids, between circulation and calm, between light and structure. Vitamin P embodies that harmony, working quietly behind the scenes to ensure that energy and color flow smoothly through the skin.

Over time, consistent use of Vitamin P transforms the complexion into one that is both vibrant and composed. Redness softens, tone evens, and the surface gains a subtle vitality that reflects balanced circulation and steady repair. It is not the loud, dramatic change of a peel or resurfacing, it is the deep, graceful strengthening that endures. In every fruit-colored serum or plant-rich formula containing bioflavonoids, there is a whisper of nature's wisdom: that protection is not resistance, but rhythm, and that beauty is not created, but cultivated in cooperation with the living world.

Vitamin-Like Nutrients

Not all nutrients that support the skin's health are classified as true vitamins, yet some perform roles so essential to cellular balance, repair, and longevity that they deserve equal reverence. These "vitamin-like" substances, Choline, Coenzyme Q10 (CoQ10), Inositol, and Lycopene, occupy a space between nutrition and energy, structure and defense. They do not fit neatly into the alphabetical canon of vitamins, but they work alongside them in the skin's intricate symphony of renewal. Together they represent the emerging frontier of esthetic science: optimizing the cell's microenvironment so that the visible skin can thrive.

Choline – The Architect of Cellular Integrity

Choline is a water-soluble compound once grouped with the B-vitamins because of its pivotal role in fat metabolism and cell membrane structure. Its story begins in the mid-1800s, when chemists first isolated it from bile, and it was later recognized as an essential nutrient by the National Academy of Medicine in 1998. Biochemically, choline is the building block of phosphatidylcholine, a key phospholipid in every cell membrane, including those of keratinocytes and fibroblasts in the skin. Without it, membranes lose fluidity, signaling falters, and cells struggle to retain moisture.

In skincare, choline's influence shows in barrier strength and hydration. Healthy phospholipid layers allow the skin to hold water efficiently and maintain suppleness. When choline intake is low, the skin often appears dull, fatigued, or unevenly textured, signs of structural fatigue rather than superficial dryness. Internally, choline aids in the transport and metabolism of lipids, preventing the buildup of fatty deposits in the liver and ensuring that essential fatty acids reach the skin where they are needed most.

Choline also plays a subtle neurochemical role: it is the precursor to acetylcholine, a neurotransmitter that regulates muscle tone and communication between nerves and skin cells. This connection hints at why choline may help preserve firmness and responsiveness, qualities that decline with age. Nutritional sources include eggs, soybeans, and sunflower lecithin, while topical formulations often use phosphatidylcholine as both an emulsifier and an active ingredient. When applied to the skin, it supports lipid barrier recovery and enhances the penetration of other nutrients. In professional use, phosphatidylcholine can be found in hydrating serums and post-peel recovery creams, where it smooths texture and replenishes moisture without heaviness.

Coenzyme Q10 – The Cellular Powerhouse

If choline builds the house, Coenzyme Q10 (CoQ10) provides the electricity that keeps it running. Also known as ubiquinone, CoQ10 was discovered in 1957 by Dr. Frederick Crane and earned its name from its ubiquity; it exists in every living cell. Within the mitochondria, CoQ10 acts as an electron carrier in the respiratory chain, converting nutrients into adenosine triphosphate (ATP), the energy currency of life. The skin, which renews itself continuously, depends heavily on this energy to fuel repair and regeneration.

As we age, CoQ10 levels decline, leading to slower cellular turnover and diminished resilience. Environmental stressors such as UV exposure further deplete it, creating a feedback loop of fatigue and oxidative damage. Topically replenished CoQ10 restores vitality to aging skin by increasing mitochondrial efficiency and neutralizing free radicals generated by sunlight and pollution. In this way, it acts as both an energy booster and an antioxidant.

Several clinical studies confirm its efficacy. A 2015 Biofactors study found that topical application of CoQ10 improved skin smoothness and reduced wrinkle depth by 17% after six weeks, primarily through enhanced collagen synthesis and antioxidant defense. Its fat-soluble nature allows it to integrate easily into the lipid layers of the epidermis, where it guards against peroxidation and reinforces barrier stability. When combined with Vitamins E and C, CoQ10 creates a potent triad that prevents premature aging by protecting both mitochondrial DNA and the surrounding cell membranes.

For estheticians, CoQ10 is a rejuvenating ally, particularly in treatments aimed at restoring radiance or counteracting fatigue. Applied through massage or incorporated into serums, it lends the skin a luminous, energized quality, the visible expression of revived cellular metabolism. Over time, regular use helps the skin regain its youthful rhythm, appearing firmer, smoother, and more awake.

Inositol – The Balancer of Flow and Calm

Inositol, sometimes referred to as "Vitamin B8," is another vitamin-like nutrient integral to skin harmony. Discovered in the mid-19th century as part of muscle tissue (hence the name derived from inos, Greek for "muscle"), Inositol is a sugar-alcohol compound that functions as a cellular messenger. It helps regulate how cells respond to hormones, neurotransmitters, and nutrients.

Within the skin, Inositol contributes to lipid balance and hydration by supporting the synthesis of phosphatidylinositol, a molecule critical to the signaling pathways that control cell growth and barrier repair. It also helps regulate sebum production, making it especially useful for oily or acne-prone clients whose skin struggles to find equilibrium. By moderating the hormonal signals that trigger excess oil, Inositol brings the complexion back into balance without stripping or over-drying.

In addition, Inositol has a calming influence on the nervous system and, by extension, the skin. It supports serotonin balance, reducing stress-related inflammation and flare-ups. Clients who experience breakouts or redness during times of anxiety often respond well to products or supplements containing Inositol, which help restore both emotional and epidermal steadiness. Dietary sources include whole grains, citrus fruits, cantaloupe, and beans, while topical forms appear in hydrating tonics and balancing serums.

Clinically, Inositol has been shown to improve barrier repair and reduce transepidermal water loss by enhancing lipid synthesis in keratinocytes. When paired with Niacinamide or Panthenol, it strengthens the skin's moisture network and reduces surface roughness. For estheticians, it functions as a harmonizer, quietly adjusting what is out of sync and creating a complexion that feels grounded, soft, and balanced.

Lycopene – The Defender of Light

Where the previous nutrients focus on structure and energy, Lycopene stands as the radiant defender, a carotenoid pigment that protects the skin from light-induced aging. Discovered in tomatoes in the early 1900s, its deep red color hints at its power: the ability to absorb and neutralize singlet oxygen, one of the most destructive forms of free radicals produced by UV radiation. Among all carotenoids, Lycopene is considered one of the most potent antioxidants, outperforming even beta-carotene in quenching reactive oxygen species.

Lycopene resides within cell membranes and the lipid layers of the stratum corneum, where it acts as a natural photo-shield. It reduces oxidative stress, inhibits inflammation, and prevents the degradation of collagen caused by ultraviolet exposure. Several studies have shown that dietary or topical Lycopene can decrease erythema and improve skin texture. A 2017 British Journal of Dermatology study found that participants who consumed tomato extract containing Lycopene daily for 12 weeks exhibited 40% less UV-induced damage and smoother, more even-toned skin.

Topically, Lycopene is oil-soluble and best delivered through lipid carriers such as squalane or jojoba. Its brilliant pigment also imparts a subtle golden-rosy hue to formulations, often used in brightening oils and antioxidant serums. When combined with Vitamins C and E, Lycopene creates a protective matrix that reinforces both the hydrophilic and lipophilic defenses of the skin, an antioxidant network that mirrors the plant's own survival strategy.

For estheticians, Lycopene-rich products are invaluable in summer or in clients exposed to high levels of environmental stress. Used before and after sun exposure, it helps preserve firmness and reduce redness, allowing the complexion to maintain its natural equilibrium. Over time, consistent use enhances luminosity, not the artificial gleam of resurfacing, but the deep internal glow of a skin that is both protected and nourished.

Each of these nutrients, Choline, CoQ10, Inositol, and Lycopene, operates on a different level of the skin's hierarchy, yet together they form a holistic network of vitality. Choline builds structure and barrier integrity; CoQ10 energizes and protects the mitochondria; Inositol harmonizes signaling and balance; and Lycopene defends against light and oxidation. They represent four aspects of a single truth: that beauty is sustained not only by repair, but by rhythm.

Pro Tip: Combine a CoQ10-enriched serum with a Lycopene facial oil for daytime antioxidant defense, then apply a phosphatidylcholine-rich moisturizer at night to rebuild the barrier. Adding an Inositol supplement or infusion can further balance sebum and hydration, supporting a 24-hour cycle of energy and calm.

Clinical Insight: A 2021 review in Nutrients found that supplementation with CoQ10, Lycopene, and Choline for 12 weeks improved skin elasticity by 18% and reduced oxidative markers by 25%, while Inositol decreased sebum oxidation and improved hydration in oily skin types, confirming the synergistic value of these vitamin-like compounds.

Philosophically, these nutrients embody the bridge between science and subtlety. They work not by forcing change, but by teaching the skin to remember its original intelligence, to circulate energy, retain moisture, and reflect light naturally. They show that health is not static but rhythmic, powered by continual exchange: between membrane and mitochondrion, pigment and photon, nourishment and renewal.

Over time, consistent use of vitamin-like nutrients transforms the complexion into one that hums with quiet vitality. Lines soften, tone brightens, and the skin behaves with youthful responsiveness. It is not a miracle of surface transformation but of restored dialogue within the cell, a conversation between energy, structure, and light. These nutrients remind us that skincare is not just chemistry; it is choreography, and the most beautiful skin is that which moves in harmony with its own living rhythm.

Conclusion

Every nutrient we've explored speaks to the skin in its own dialect: Vitamin A commands renewal, Vitamin C shines light through collagen, Vitamin D builds strength from shadow, Vitamin E guards the gate against time, Vitamin K closes the circle of repair. The B vitamins hum together in quiet industry, generating energy and balance. And beyond them, the vitamin-like nutrients, CoQ10, Choline, Inositol, Lycopene, work in subtler ways, orchestrating harmony beneath the visible surface. The more we understand these messengers, the more clearly we see that the skin is not a passive canvas but an intelligent organ in constant conversation with its environment.

The skin is alive with memory. It remembers every sunbeam, every nutrient, every night of rest or neglect. It remembers the difference between deficiency and abundance, between depletion and renewal. And yet, it never holds grudges. Give it what it needs, time, nourishment, oxygen, vitamins, and it begins again. That is the miracle we call rejuvenation. True skincare is not manipulation; it is cooperation with this intelligence. It means understanding how each nutrient directs the symphony of growth and decay that keeps us looking human, radiant, and alive.

Through each chapter, a pattern emerges. Vitamins are not isolated miracles; they are interdependent. None can perform its function without the others. Vitamin C needs Vitamin P to hold its power. Vitamin A needs Zinc to activate its message. Vitamin D needs Magnesium to convert sunlight into strength. Vitamin K restores balance after Vitamin E has shielded the cells from harm. These connections reveal the skin's deeper truth: beauty is not a product of dominance but of relationship. When one nutrient is missing, the others labor harder. When all are present in harmony, the result is not only health but presence, a glow that comes from coherence.

The practice of esthetics, at its highest level, is an act of translation. The esthetician becomes a bridge between chemistry and consciousness, reading the silent messages of the skin and responding with precision, empathy, and respect. Knowing which vitamin to apply or suggest is not guesswork, it is literacy. It is learning to read the fine print of the body's needs. To see dehydration not merely as dryness, but as a signal of disrupted lipid synthesis; to see dullness not as a flaw, but as a symptom of oxidative fatigue. Vitamins are the alphabet by which we decode those signals and respond in kind.

Science gives us the mechanisms, but intuition gives us the music. This is what separates a technician from an artist. To understand that Vitamin C's glow is not only chemical but symbolic, the embodiment of light made tangible. That Vitamin A's peeling is not damage but transformation. That Vitamin K's calming effect mirrors the process of forgiveness after trauma. In this sense, every treatment becomes both a biochemical and spiritual ritual, a rebalancing of the seen and unseen forces that shape the skin's story.

As we move deeper into an era of technology-driven beauty, LED therapy, peptides, growth factors, bioidentical hormones, it becomes even more essential to remember that these tools rest upon the same foundation as they always have: the body's natural intelligence. No machine can replace the laws of cellular nutrition. The future of skincare will not belong to those who use the most advanced devices, but to those who understand how energy, oxygen, and nutrients sustain life at its most delicate interface. Vitamins remain the original anti-aging technology, timeless, adaptive, and universally available.

The more we study the chemistry of the skin, the more spiritual it becomes. To watch a damaged barrier rebuild after weeks of nourishment is to witness faith made visible. To see pigmentation fade as antioxidant levels rise is to understand that clarity begins with balance. The skin, like the self, cannot be rushed. It listens only to consistency, patience, and respect. Each vitamin we've studied reminds us of this truth: repair is not a single act but a rhythm. The esthetician's task is not to force that rhythm but to guide it, to know when to stimulate, when to soothe, when to wait.

In a world saturated with instant results and surface perfection, there is power in remembering that true radiance is cumulative. It builds slowly, cell by cell, nourished by the quiet constancy of nutrients doing their work unseen. Vitamins teach us that beauty is not the absence of flaws but the presence of vitality. A face that glows is one that participates fully in its own healing. It is alive to the conversation between body and world.

Glossary

Absorption

The process by which nutrients or topical ingredients pass through the skin barrier or digestive tract into circulation or cellular layers. Effective absorption depends on molecular size, solubility, and the integrity of the skin's lipid barrier.

Acid Mantle

A slightly acidic film on the skin's surface composed of sebum, sweat, and natural acids that helps maintain microbial balance. When disrupted, it can lead to irritation, dehydration, and increased sensitivity.

Amino Acids

The organic compounds that form proteins such as collagen, elastin, and keratin—core building blocks of skin tissue. They also contribute to hydration and repair by forming part of the skin's Natural Moisturizing Factor (NMF).

Antioxidant

A molecule that neutralizes free radicals before they can damage cellular DNA, lipids, and proteins. Antioxidants like Vitamins C and E are vital for slowing visible aging and preventing inflammation.

Ascorbic Acid

The pure, biologically active form of Vitamin C known for its role in collagen synthesis and brightening. It helps reverse oxidative damage while promoting firmer, more even-toned skin.

ATP (Adenosine Triphosphate)

The body's universal energy currency, produced by mitochondria through cellular respiration. Every act of repair, renewal, and regeneration in the skin relies on ATP for fuel.

Autophagy

A natural cellular process in which damaged or aging components are broken down and recycled. In the skin, autophagy supports longevity and resilience, reducing visible signs of stress and fatigue.

Barrier Function

The skin's ability to retain water and block external irritants, microbes, and toxins. A strong barrier depends on balanced lipids, ceramides, and natural oils.

Beta-Carotene

An orange-red pigment found in plants that serves as a precursor to Vitamin A. It provides antioxidant protection against UV-induced oxidative stress and supports healthy cell renewal.

Bioavailability

The percentage of a nutrient or ingredient that reaches its target site in an active form. High bioavailability ensures that applied vitamins or supplements produce visible and measurable effects in the skin.

Bioflavonoids (Vitamin P)

Plant compounds that strengthen capillaries, enhance Vitamin C absorption, and reduce inflammation. They are found in citrus fruits, green tea, and berries, offering both vascular and antioxidant support.

Biotin (Vitamin B7)

A water-soluble B-vitamin that supports keratin production for strong hair, nails, and skin. Deficiency often results in dryness, scaling, or brittle nails.

Botanical Extract

A concentrated preparation derived from flowers, roots, or leaves that delivers phytonutrients to the skin. Each extract has its own biochemical profile and can calm, brighten, or protect depending on its source.

Buffer

A stabilizing agent that maintains the correct pH level of skincare formulas. Buffers prevent irritation caused by highly acidic or alkaline ingredients.

Capillaries

Tiny blood vessels beneath the skin that supply nutrients and oxygen while removing waste. Their fragility can lead to redness or visible veins, which nutrients like Vitamin K help repair.

Carotenoids

A group of natural pigments that protect plants and skin cells from oxidative damage. They give fruits and vegetables their red, orange, and yellow hues and act as antioxidants when consumed or applied topically.

Ceramides

Waxy lipid molecules naturally found in the skin that form part of its protective barrier. They prevent transepidermal water loss and keep the surface soft, hydrated, and resilient.

Chelation

A process in which minerals or metals bind with another molecule to improve stability or eliminate toxicity. In skincare, chelators keep products stable and help detoxify environmental metals from the skin.

Choline

A vitamin-like nutrient vital for building healthy cell membranes and metabolizing fats. It supports smooth texture and moisture retention through its role in phospholipid synthesis.

Collagen

The primary structural protein that maintains firmness and elasticity within the dermis. Collagen breakdown leads to wrinkles and sagging, while Vitamins C and A stimulate its renewal.

Coenzyme Q10 (CoQ10)

A powerful antioxidant and energy carrier present in every living cell. It energizes skin cells, reduces oxidative stress, and improves visible signs of aging.

Comedone

A clogged pore resulting from trapped sebum and dead cells; open comedones are blackheads, closed are whiteheads. Maintaining exfoliation and sebum balance helps prevent their formation.

Cytokines

Protein messengers that coordinate immune and inflammatory responses in the skin. They regulate healing but can also trigger chronic redness when overproduced.

Dehydration

A temporary condition in which the skin lacks water but not necessarily oil. It causes tightness, dullness, and fine lines that improve with humectants like hyaluronic acid.

Dermis

The middle layer of the skin that houses collagen, elastin, nerves, and blood vessels. It provides strength and nourishment to the epidermis above it.

Desquamation

The natural process by which dead cells are shed from the skin's surface. This cycle keeps the complexion smooth, bright, and receptive to nutrients.

Diffusion

The passive movement of molecules from an area of high concentration to low concentration. It is one of the fundamental processes through which ingredients penetrate the skin.

DNA (Deoxyribonucleic Acid)

The molecule carrying genetic instructions for cellular growth and repair. Vitamins, minerals, and antioxidants protect DNA from UV-induced mutations that accelerate aging.

Dosage

The specific amount or concentration of a nutrient required to achieve a désired effect. Proper dosing ensures efficacy without irritation or toxicity.

Epidermis

The outermost layer of the skin composed primarily of keratinocytes. It provides protection, regulates hydration, and continuously renews itself every 28–40 days.

Erythema

Redness of the skin due to increased blood flow, often a result of inflammation or irritation. It is both a sign of healing and a symptom of stress.

Essential Fatty Acids (EFAs)

Healthy fats such as omega-3 and omega-6 that the body cannot synthesize. They maintain barrier integrity, reduce inflammation, and support supple texture.

Exfoliation

The removal of dead surface cells through chemical or mechanical means. It encourages renewal, enhances absorption, and improves clarity.

Extracellular Matrix (ECM)

A complex network of collagen, elastin, and glycoproteins that provide support and structure to the dermis. Vitamins, minerals, and peptides help preserve its resilience.

Fat-Soluble Vitamins

Vitamins A, D, E, and K that dissolve in fats and are stored in the body's tissues. They provide long-term protection, regeneration, and repair within the skin.

Folate (Vitamin B9)

A B-vitamin essential for DNA synthesis and tissue growth. Adequate folate helps maintain smooth, even-toned skin by supporting cell turnover.

Free Radicals

Unstable molecules produced by pollution, UV light, or stress that damage skin cells. Antioxidants neutralize these radicals to prevent premature aging.

Fibroblast

A connective tissue cell responsible for producing collagen, elastin, and hyaluronic acid. Stimulating fibroblast activity is the goal of many anti-aging treatments.

Glycation

The process where sugar molecules bind to proteins, forming rigid structures called AGEs (Advanced Glycation End-products). This stiffens collagen and accelerates wrinkling.

Glutathione

A master antioxidant naturally produced in the body that detoxifies cells and lightens hyperpigmentation. It is crucial in skin brightening and immune defense.

Gamma-Linolenic Acid (GLA)

An omega-6 fatty acid found in evening primrose and borage oil. It calms inflammation, restores moisture, and strengthens the skin barrier.

Hyaluronic Acid

A molecule that binds up to 1,000 times its weight in water, delivering deep hydration and plumpness. Naturally present in the skin, it declines with age, leading to dryness and fine lines.

Hormonal Acne

Breakouts triggered by hormonal fluctuations affecting sebum production and inflammation. Balancing internal health and using calming, non-comedogenic ingredients helps control it.

Hydration

The water content within the skin's layers that determines softness, suppleness, and elasticity. Proper hydration balances oil production and supports all cellular functions.

Hydrolysis

A chemical reaction that breaks larger molecules into smaller, more absorbable units using water. It is used in skincare to make proteins like collagen more bioavailable.

Hyperpigmentation

Excess melanin production resulting in dark spots or uneven tone. It often follows inflammation, UV exposure, or hormonal changes.

Inflammation

The body's natural response to injury or stress, characterized by redness, swelling, and heat. While essential for healing, chronic inflammation leads to aging and sensitivity.

Inositol

A vitamin-like compound that helps regulate lipid balance and hormone signaling. It restores equilibrium to oily or reactive skin, promoting calm and clarity.

Isoflavones

Plant-derived compounds that mimic estrogen and stimulate collagen production. Found in soy, they help maintain skin thickness and elasticity after hormonal decline.

Isomer

A molecule with the same formula but a different structure, sometimes altering biological activity. In skincare, one isomer can be more effective or stable than another.

Jojoba Oil

A liquid wax that closely resembles human sebum, making it highly biocompatible. It balances oil levels and supports barrier repair without clogging pores.

Keratin

A strong fibrous protein forming the structure of skin, hair, and nails. Its integrity determines smoothness and resilience.

Keratinocytes

The predominant cells of the epidermis responsible for producing keratin. Their lifecycle drives renewal and barrier strength.

Kojic Acid

A natural compound derived from fungi that inhibits tyrosinase, reducing pigmentation. It is often used in brightening and spot-correcting formulas.

L-Ascorbic Acid

The most potent form of Vitamin C used in professional skincare. It stimulates collagen synthesis and lightens hyperpigmentation through antioxidant action.

Lactic Acid

An alpha-hydroxy acid that gently exfoliates while increasing hydration. Suitable for sensitive skin, it promotes smooth texture and brightness.

Lecithin

A phospholipid used as an emulsifier and moisturizer in skincare. It supports lipid barrier recovery and helps ingredients penetrate more effectively.

Lipid Barrier

The outermost layer of the skin composed of fats, cholesterol, and ceramides. It keeps moisture in and pollutants out, acting as the body's frontline defense.

Lycopene

A deep red carotenoid antioxidant found in tomatoes and watermelon. It shields skin from UV-induced oxidative stress and enhances overall radiance.

Macronutrients

Proteins, fats, and carbohydrates required in large amounts for growth and energy. Skin health relies on balanced intake to maintain structure and hydration.

Magnesium

A mineral that activates hundreds of enzymatic reactions, including Vitamin D metabolism. It helps calm inflammation and supports cellular repair.

Melanin

The pigment produced by melanocytes that determines skin color and protects against UV radiation. Balanced melanin production results in even tone and natural defense.

Microcirculation

The flow of blood through the smallest capillaries in the dermis. Good microcirculation ensures oxygen and nutrients reach the skin efficiently.

Micronutrients

Vitamins and minerals required in trace amounts for enzymatic activity. They regulate everything from collagen synthesis to immune defense.

Mitochondria

The "powerhouses" of the cell responsible for generating ATP energy. Their efficiency declines with age, contributing to slower healing and dullness.

Moisturization

The process of increasing and retaining water and lipids in the skin. It restores comfort, prevents TEWL, and enhances elasticity.

Niacinamide (Vitamin B3)

A multitasking vitamin that improves barrier strength, brightens tone, and reduces redness. It also regulates sebum production and repairs oxidative stress.

Neuropeptides

Messenger molecules that influence how the skin responds to stress and movement. They are used in anti-aging products to relax expression lines and promote regeneration.

NMF (Natural Moisturizing Factor)

A complex of amino acids, lactic acid, and urea that naturally hydrate the skin. It maintains softness and elasticity by binding water within the stratum corneum.

Occlusive

An ingredient that forms a physical barrier on the surface to prevent water loss. Examples include petrolatum, beeswax, and certain plant oils.

Oxygenation

The process of delivering oxygen to cells for energy and repair. Well-oxygenated skin appears brighter, more even, and youthful.

Oxidation

A chemical reaction involving oxygen that can degrade fats, DNA, or vitamins. In skincare, antioxidants prevent oxidation to preserve both formulas and skin health.

Panthenol (Vitamin B5)

A humectant that attracts moisture and promotes healing. It soothes irritation and supports barrier recovery after exfoliation or environmental stress.

pH Balance

The measure of acidity or alkalinity of the skin, ideally between 4.5 and 5.5. Maintaining this range prevents bacterial growth and supports barrier function.

Peptides

Short chains of amino acids that signal the skin to produce collagen or repair damage. They act as biological messengers that stimulate youthful activity.

Phosphatidylcholine

A lipid molecule derived from choline that supports cell membranes and nutrient delivery. In skincare, it stabilizes emulsions and enhances penetration.

Photodamage

Skin damage resulting from UV radiation that accelerates aging and pigmentation. Antioxidants, sunscreen, and Vitamins C and E prevent and repair this harm.

Phytochemicals

Bioactive plant compounds that provide antioxidant, anti-inflammatory, and protective effects. They include flavonoids, terpenes, and polyphenols used in botanical skincare.

Pigmentation

The natural coloring of the skin caused by melanin distribution. Uneven pigmentation results from inflammation, hormonal changes, or UV exposure.

Provitamin

A precursor molecule that converts into an active vitamin within the body. Beta-carotene, for instance, becomes Vitamin A when metabolized.

Quercetin

A potent bioflavonoid found in apples and onions that reduces inflammation and strengthens vessels. It enhances antioxidant defenses and soothes sensitivity.

Retinol (Vitamin A)

A derivative of Vitamin A that accelerates cell turnover and collagen renewal. It improves texture, tone, and fine lines through controlled regeneration.

Riboflavin (Vitamin B2)

A B-vitamin that supports tissue repair and energy production. It contributes to healthy mucous membranes and vibrant skin tone.

Rosacea

A chronic vascular condition marked by redness, flushing, and visible blood vessels. Managing inflammation and strengthening capillaries are key to controlling it.

Rutin

A citrus bioflavonoid that enhances Vitamin C stability and improves circulation. It reduces redness and supports capillary strength in sensitive skin.

Sebum

The oily substance produced by sebaceous glands that lubricates and protects the skin. Balanced sebum levels maintain softness while preventing dehydration.

Selenium

A trace mineral that neutralizes oxidative stress and supports Vitamin E's antioxidant activity. It helps prevent inflammation and premature aging.

Sensitization

A process by which the skin becomes increasingly reactive to ingredients or environmental triggers. Once sensitized, the skin requires barrier repair and reduced stimulation.

Serum

A concentrated, lightweight formula designed to deliver high doses of active ingredients. Serums penetrate quickly, targeting specific concerns like aging, pigmentation, or dehydration.

Squalane

A hydrogenated form of squalene that mimics natural skin lipids. It provides moisture and protection without greasiness or comedogenic effects.

Stratum Corneum

The outermost layer of the epidermis composed of dead cells and lipids. It acts as the skin's armor, protecting deeper layers from dehydration and toxins.

Telangiectasia

Small, dilated blood vessels visible near the skin's surface, often caused by chronic inflammation or sun exposure. Treatments with Vitamin K or bioflavonoids can help reduce their appearance.

Topical Application

Applying a substance directly to the skin for local absorption. This method allows vitamins and actives to work where they're needed most.

Trace Elements

Micronutrients such as zinc, copper, and selenium needed in very small amounts for enzymatic and structural support. Even minimal deficiencies can affect collagen production and immunity.

Transepidermal Water Loss (TEWL)

The process of water evaporating through the epidermis into the air. Measuring TEWL helps determine barrier health and hydration needs.

Tyrosinase

An enzyme that catalyzes the production of melanin in skin cells. Inhibiting tyrosinase is the goal of many brightening and depigmenting treatments.

Ubiquinone

Another name for Coenzyme Q10, a vitamin-like antioxidant that energizes cells and protects against oxidative damage. It supports mitochondrial efficiency and firmness.

Ultraviolet Radiation (UV)

Invisible rays from the sun divided into UVA and UVB, both of which cause DNA damage and premature aging. Regular sunscreen use and antioxidant defense are essential to mitigate UV harm.

Vasodilation

The widening of blood vessels that increases circulation and nutrient delivery to tissues. While beneficial for healing, excessive vasodilation can cause flushing or redness.

Vitamin-Like Nutrients

Compounds that perform vitamin-like roles but are not officially classified as vitamins, such as CoQ10, Inositol, and Lycopene. They contribute to energy, balance, and antioxidant protection within the skin.

Further Reading

Healthline: "The Benefits — and Limits — of Vitamin A for Your Skin"

https://www.healthline.com/health/vitamin-a-for-skin

American Academy of Dermatology: "Acne Clinical Guideline"

https://www.aad.org/member/clinical-quality/guidelines/acne

Mayo Clinic: "Wrinkle Creams: Your Guide to Younger-looking Skin"

https://www.mayoclinic.org/diseases-conditions/wrinkles/in-depth/wrinkle-creams/art-20047463

Healthline: "Everything You Should Know About Niacinamide"

https://www.healthline.com/health/beauty-skin-care/niacinamide

Susan G. Komen Foundation: "Niacinamide" https://www.komen.org/breast-cancer/survivorship/complementary-therapies/niacinamide/

Marie Claire: "Niacinamide for Acne: What to Know, According to Dermatologists" https://www.marieclaire.com/beauty/niacinamide-for-acne/

Medical News Today: "List of the Best Vitamins for Skin" https://www.medicalnewstoday.com/articles/324943

National Center for Biotechnology Information: "Niacinamide: A B Vitamin that Improves Aging Facial Skin Appearance"

https://pubmed.ncbi.nlm.nih.gov/16029679/

Medical News Today: "What You Need to Know About Acne"

https://www.medicalnewstoday.com/articles/107146

Dermatologic Therapy: "The Role of Nicotinamide in Acne Treatment" https://pubmed.ncbi.nlm.nih.gov/28220628/

Wiley Online Library: "A Comparative Study of the Effects of Retinol and Retinoic Acid on Histological, Molecular, and Clinical Properties of Human Skin"

https://onlinelibrary.wiley.com/doi/full/10.1111/jocd.12193

Nutrients: "The Roles of Vitamin C in Skin Health" https://www.ncbi.nlm.nih.gov/pmc/articles/PMC5579659/

Indian Dermatology Online Journal: "Vitamin C in Dermatology"
https://www.ncbi.nlm.nih.gov/pmc/articles/PMC3673383/

Healthline: "The Benefits of a Vitamin C Facial for Bright, Smooth Skin"
https://www.healthline.com/health/beauty-skin-care/vitamin-c-facial#benefits-for-your-face

Vogue: "How to Use Vitamin C in Your Skin-Care Routine Correctly, According to the Experts"
https://www.vogue.com/article/how-to-use-vitamin-c-in-your-skin-care-routine-correctly

Healthline: "11 Reasons to Add Vitamin C Serum to Your Skin Care Routine"
https://www.healthline.com/health/beauty-skin-care/vitamin-c-serum-benefits

Drug Delivery: "Magnesium Ascorbyl Phosphate Vesicular Carriers for Topical Delivery; Preparation, In-vitro and Ex-vivo Evaluation, Factorial Optimization and Clinical Assessment in Melasma Patients" https://www.ncbi.nlm.nih.gov/pmc/articles/PMC9040897/

Journal of Clinical and Aesthetic Dermatology: "Topical Vitamin C and the Skin: Mechanisms of Action and Clinical Applications" https://www.ncbi.nlm.nih.gov/pmc/articles/PMC5605218/

Harvard T.H. Chan School of Public Health: "Vitamin D and Health"
https://www.hsph.harvard.edu/nutritionsource/vitamin-d/

Medical News Today: "What are the Health Benefits of Vitamin D?"
https://www.medicalnewstoday.com/articles/161618

Healthline: "The Great Sunscreen Debate: Vitamin D vs. Skin Cancer"

https://www.healthline.com/health-news/sunscreen-vitamin-d-deficiency

American Osteopathic Association: "Widespread Vitamin D Deficiency Likely Due to Sunscreen Use, Increase of Chronic Diseases"

https://osteopathic.org/2017/05/01/widespread-vitamin-d-deficiency-likely-due-to-sunscreen-use-increase-of-chronic-diseases/

Skin Cancer Foundation: "Sun Protection and Vitamin D" https://www.skincancer.org/blog/sun-protection-and-vitamin-d/

Indian Dermatology Online Journal: "Vitamin E in dermatology" https://www.ncbi.nlm.nih.gov/pmc/articles/PMC4976416/

Dermatological Surgery: "Vitamin E: Critical Review of its Current Use in Cosmetic and Clinical Dermatology" https://pubmed.ncbi.nlm.nih.gov/16029671/

Molecular Aspects of Medicine: "Vitamin E in Human Skin: Organ-Specific Physiology and Considerations for its Use in Dermatology" https://pubmed.ncbi.nlm.nih.gov/17719081/

Healthline: Vitamin E and Your Skin, Friends Through Food

https://www.healthline.com/health/vitamin-e-for-skin

The Journal of Clinical and Aesthetic Dermatology: "Skin Anti-aging Strategies" https://www.ncbi.nlm.nih.gov/pmc/articles/PMC3583892/

Cutaneous and Ocular Toxicology: "Evaluation of Serum Vitamins A and E and Zinc Levels According to the Severity of Acne Vulgaris" https://pubmed.ncbi.nlm.nih.gov/23826827/

Indian Journal of Pharmacology: "Wound Healing Effects of Topical Vitamin K" https://pubmed.ncbi.nlm.nih.gov/31142943/

Healthline: "The 4 Best Vitamins for Your Skin" https://www.healthline.com/health/4-best-vitamins-for-skin

Real Simple: "Is Vitamin K the Secret to Anti-Aging? Here's What You Need to Know" https://www.realsimple.com/beauty-fashion/skincare/anti-aging/vitamin-k-benefits

Healthline "Vitamin F Health Benefits"

https://www.healthline.com/nutrition/vitamin-f

Cleveland Clinic: "Vitamin F"

https://my.clevelandclinic.org/health/articles/23109-vitamin-f

Medical News Today: "Vitamin F: What it is, and why we need it"

https://www.medicalnewstoday.com/articles/vitamin-f

European Journal of Pharmaceutics and Biopharmaceutics: "The Clinical Efficacy of Cosmeceutical Application of Liquid Crystalline Nanostructured Dispersions of Alpha Lipoic Acid as Anti-Wrinkle"

https://pubmed.ncbi.nlm.nih.gov/24056055/

NSSG Club: "Do you know about vitamin P and its benefits?"

https://www.nssgclub.com/en/beauty/33407/benefici-vitamina-p#:~:text=It%20can%20help%20reduce%20redness,those%20prone%20to%20skin%20problems.&text=Another%20benefit%20of%20vitamin%20P%20is%20its%20antioxidant%20effect.

Reviva Labs: "Vitamin P: Good News for Spider Veins and Redness"

https://www.revivalabs.com/vitamin-p-good-news-for-spider-veins-and-redness/

Daily Skin Care: "Vitamin P for Skincare"

http://www.dailyskincare.net/skin-care/vitamin-p-for-skin-care/33/

www.ingramcontent.com/pod-product-compliance
Lightning Source LLC
Chambersburg PA
CBHW070810260726
48660CB00005B/1798